Strength Training for Women over 40

The Complete Guide to Strength Training for Women over 40

Nancy Petersen

Copyright © 2023 by Nancy Petersen

All rights reserved. No part of this publication may be reproduced, distributed, or transmitted in any form or by any means, including photocopying, recording, or other electronic or mechanical methods, without the prior written permission of the publisher, except in the case of brief quotations embodied in critical reviews and certain other noncommercial uses permitted by copyright law.

Table of Contents

Introduction -- 4

What is Strength Training? -- 5

Why You Shouldn't Avoid Exercise ---------------------------------- 9

Why is Cardio Exercise a Waste of Time? ------------------------- 23

Will You Need a Lot of Workout Equipment? -------------------- 29

Practice the Moves --- 37

The Fundamentals of Strength Training -------------------------- 59

The Extreme Workout Plan --- 72

Important Nutrients -- 82

The importance of consistency -------------------------------------- 94

Conclusion -- 101

Introduction

Did you know that at the age of 40, you can lose a pound of muscle per year? I believed you should be aware. When it comes to losing muscle as we get older, the proverb "use it or lose it" is especially accurate. After a person is 30 years old, they typically begin to naturally lose muscle mass, and as time goes on, this loss accelerates. As a consequence, you become less flexible and more prone to accidents as your body ages and your muscles start to lose strength.

Most of us live contemporary, technologically advanced lives. We no longer put the same amount of strain on our bodies as our forefathers did. Almost everything we do is done by machines. Because it is no longer being used, our bodies have reacted by eroding our muscular mass and strength. Because of this, persons who continue to be physically inactive age more rapidly than those who continue to be physically active.

According to research, losing muscle has a negative impact on your body and general health. In addition to others, it is linked to fat gain, sluggish metabolism, physical dysfunction, joint and back pain, and bone loss.

Most of us are concerned that as we age, we will become weak, helpless, and unable to take care of ourselves. Also, we are pondering in silence how our later years will proceed. As the years go by, we tend to lose all hope for our overall health. Don't give up. It's still possible. You may take action to counteract Mother Nature. You can, indeed. Strength training, not witchcraft or anything else associated with black magic.

Several medical and scientific studies have shown that strength training is the most crucial action you can take to reverse the aging process and say goodbye to the health issues that come with it, as well as to stop muscle loss and slow down the aging process. Learn more about strength training before continuing.

What is Strength Training?

Several people confuse strength training with bodybuilding, but they are not the same thing. Strength training, often known as resistance training, is the use of your own body weight, free weights (such as dumbbells, barbells, and kettlebells), or weight from gym equipment to do exercises that develop skeletal muscular strength and endurance. It is necessary for the muscles to struggle against and conquer the weights. You raise the weights in opposition to the downward force exerted by gravity.

The purpose of strength training, particularly for those in their 40s and older, is to increase general body strength in order to become more physically capable of maintaining functional mobility and making everyday tasks more doable. It also helps you keep active and healthy regardless of your age.

Also, strength training increases muscles, but not at the same pace as bodybuilding. Bodybuilding is mainly associated with competitive exhibits, and many "bodybuilders" merely train out to achieve the sort of body that would look good on stage. This is a difficult sport to master since it is difficult to maintain a tight diet when bulking and cutting.

Overall, bodybuilding, like any other professional activity, has nothing to do with health. I think you now understand the distinction.

Whether your aim is to grow muscle or strength, you'll discover that both need comparable forms of exercise - the difference is in the number of repetitions you perform, the weights you use, and the rest period between sets. This will be covered in further depth in Chapter 5.

Misconceptions About Strength Training Among People Over 40

Strength training is one of the most misunderstood areas of fitness among those over the age of 40. This is due to common misunderstandings about strength training and aging that have crept into our culture. Most people over the age of 40 believe that: It is too late to begin strength training They will injure themselves as they exercise due to their age They can't move and lift weights as they did in their 20s Walking or cardio is sufficient for them They have a weak heart and joints, so they can't withstand high-intensity exercises Staying sedentary is the best way to prevent falls and injuries

These misunderstandings are what prevent many individuals over the age of 40 from reaping the advantages of strength training. Although many people over the age of 40 are drawn to strength training because of reports of improved bone health, increased independence and flexibility, reduced risk of osteoporosis, increased stamina, reduced depression, weight loss, and so on, they are unable to exercise because of their concerns about these myths. This book dispels these myths and offers you with genuine information regarding strength training after the age of 40.
Aging does not have to be associated with a reduction in health; rather, it is associated with a decline in our ability to adapt to change, sickness, and damage. And this is something over which we have influence and control. Strength training may be able to solve this condition. It's never too late to get in shape, whether you've been a fitness fanatic for decades or are new to strength training. Just following the strength training exercise routine in this book can help you grow strength and muscle regardless of your age.

Some individuals are afraid about having to spend a lot of time lifting pricey gym weights or paying expensive gym membership fees. To be clear, you do not need to workout for hours every day for the rest of your life to get the advantages of strength training.

A couple of times a week for roughly two or three months, 30 minutes of good strength training exercise can reverse up to 10-30 years of loss in strength and function. You also do not have to worry about acquiring costly gym equipments and equipment or paying monthly costs.

You may exercise anywhere without or with fewer gym equipment and yet get the same advantages as individuals who exercise in gyms. Do you want to know how? Don't be concerned. Just keep reading. This book will teach you how to accomplish it.

According to studies, exercise and a healthy diet are important components in obtaining excellent health and wellbeing, particularly beyond the age of 40. According to research, millions of individuals throughout the world will become feeble as they age owing to serious loss of muscular mass and strength. The good news is that you don't have to be one of them.

There are steps you may do to assist avoid or reverse the problem. We are fortunate to live in an age when we can get all of the knowledge and information we need to solve certain challenges. That is why I am sharing my expertise with you. I will provide you all the knowledge you need to be healthy, strong, and fit.

Knowing what I know about fitness and having over 20 years of research expertise on matters related to fitness, health, nutrition, and wellness, I must tell you that there are no unique items for boosting muscle mass and strength or antiaging. Anybody attempting to offer you such things is attempting to defraud you! Strength training is required to have a strong, attractive, and healthy physique.

I researched numerous fitness principles and applied what I learned to my personal training regimen as well as the routines of my friends. I've worked with hundreds of folks to help them achieve their desired body shape and stamina. Believe it or not, I recommend strength training activities to every single individual I assist reach their fitness objectives, regardless of age, size, shape, or ability. I like inspiring people and have a general interest in health and fitness.

I've tried everything from gym-focused heavy weights to cardio-focused light weights, at-home exercises, structured courses, cycling, yoga, HIIT, whole body, core strength, and dance. This has given me ample experience in the field of health and fitness. I'll tell you right now that there is no secret recipe to fitness achievement that the experts are keeping hidden from the general public. It's simple: exercise and eat healthy.

It is essential that you check your doctor before beginning any kind of workout routine. This is significant because your doctor will be able to establish whether your body is ready for exercise and will be able to advise you on the sorts of workouts you should avoid based on your health state.

Strength training is a healthy exercise. Just identify your motivation, learn how to do the exercises properly and safely, be devoted, be consistent, and rest sufficiently to enable your muscles to heal, and you will see results.

Thus, if you're over 40 and want to seem younger, like people in their twenties, or if you want to grow muscular mass, strength, flexibility, remain healthy, and boost your self-confidence, this book is for you. It contains all of the necessary information and directions to assist you in doing so.

In the first chapter, I'll explain why you can't afford to miss workouts, particularly beyond the age of 30, and what you should do to get the most out of them. Let's get started!

Why You Shouldn't Avoid Exercise

Strength training offers benefits at any age, but it has considerably greater benefits beyond the age of 40. Aging is an unavoidable fact of life. In fact, you should be grateful that you can mature, since others may not. But, as you get older, you go through a natural process that includes a loss of many things, including muscular mass and strength, which might put you at risk of chronic diseases and a shorter lifetime. The best way to avoid this is to add strength training to your routine.

In this chapter, I'll teach you how to discover your fitness whys, talk about simple techniques to increase your willpower and inspire yourself to exercise, and examine the advantages of strength training at 40 and beyond. Continue reading!

The Advantages of Strength Training for People Over 40

Muscle mass should be maintained and rebuilt. Most individuals begin to lose muscle mass around the age of 30 and lose 3-8% every decade. As you reach 50, the drop jumps to 5–10%. (Briley, 2020). As a result, establishing a regular strength training regimen is an excellent idea. It aids in muscle maintenance and rebuilding. Yet, if nothing is done, you will have lost more than half of your muscle mass by the age of 80.

Improve your flexibility, strength, and balance. Strength training exercises improve your strength, flexibility, and posture, which aid in balance and coordination and reduce your risks of falling while walking. Flexibility requires the synchronization of various bodily components, including muscles, bones, and joints. Equilibrium is essential as we age. Other concerns, such as vision and inner ear problems, may influence our balance as we age, but if we keep our strength and range of motion, we will be less likely to lose our balance.

Encourage bone health and strength. Exercise aids in bone density maintenance and bone formation. Our bones begin to lose tissue as we age. When our bones grow brittle and readily shatter, we are more likely to experience trauma and fractures. Those who exercise consistently, regardless of age, build strong bones, tissues, and muscles, according to research. When your bones are stressed, they react by producing more cells and becoming denser. Frequent strength exercises will therefore assist you in building bone tissues and slowing the loss of bone density that occurs with aging. Enhance your brain's health. Numerous studies have shown a link between physical strength and cognitive performance in the elderly. Better cognitive capabilities result from increased physical strength. When we talk about cognitive processes, we mean brain functions like receiving, storing, processing, and utilizing information. According to Florida Atlantic University researchers, sarcopenia (the process through which individuals lose muscular mass and strength as they age) might increase the risk of cognitive function impairment (Collins, 2020).

Strength exercise is beneficial to the aging brain for a variety of reasons, including slowing the onset of brain disorders such as Alzheimer's, having neuroprotective characteristics, reducing memory loss and multitasking, and increasing brain creativity. Frequent strength training will not only help you rebuild physical strength and boost your metabolism, but it will also help you keep your brain healthy.

Encourage better sleep. Getting adequate sleep becomes more crucial as you age for your overall health and well-being. According to studies, those who exercise on a daily basis have a better sleeping pattern. Exercise helps you fall asleep faster, sleep better at night, and wake up feeling more invigorated and refreshed.

Enhance your body's lymphatic system. For example, if you have a sore throat and notice a bump on your neck, you may massage it to relieve the swelling. This occurs in your lymphatic system, which is a network of nodes that distributes lymph fluid throughout your body. Lymph fluids aid white blood cells in their battle against infections. As a result, the lymphatic system relies on bodily movement to transport lymphatic fluid throughout the body. As a result, moving your muscles helps to circulate lymphatic fluid to all regions of your body. As a result, adequate lymphatic circulation is created.

Improve your feelings. Moving your body makes you feel better. It also alleviates anxiety and despair. Strength training has been shown in studies to benefit those suffering from emotional issues. It also enables one to deal with stress. One study looked at the role of body motions in reducing anxiety. Those who exercised several times each week had better emotions than those who did not. Those who did not exercise at all had a bad attitude. As a result, exercise is critical to avoiding acute stress.

Enhance your sexual life. Exercise benefits both men and women in their sexual lives. It promotes sexual function by increasing blood flow. It also aids in the regulation of psychological elements such as mood, stress, and confidence.

Simple Strategies to Increase Willpower and Self-Control
A lack of willpower and self-control causes the majority of our harmful and negative behaviors. Because nothing undermines willpower and self-control like stress. When you are stressed, you are more likely to overeat, overspend, oversleep or undersleep, be inactive both physically and socially, and do a variety of other things that might harm your health and general well-being. Everything that creates stress depletes our willpower and impairs our ability to control ourselves. You will be able to enjoy the

maximum advantages from exercise if you exercise regularly and with discipline and self-control.

Everything that decreases stress and enhances mood also improves our willpower and self-control. These are some strategies for reducing stress and increasing willpower and self-control: Workout on a regular basis. Exercise is the most effective approach for us to increase our self-control in all parts of our lives. This is the "quick remedy" for willpower for those seeking it. Regular exercise, according to research, decreases stress, sadness, anxiety, food and drug cravings, and enhances mood and brain function. Exercise has an immediate influence on willpower. Again, it doesn't take much to increase your willpower. In fact, studies suggest that only five minutes of low-intensity exercise may provide significant advantages. Even though it appears little, whatever workout you do restores your willpower and vitality. Thus, the next time you're weary, unmotivated, or short on time to exercise, consider the broader picture.

Get some more rest. If you don't get enough sleep, you're more likely to get agitated and fail to maintain your good behaviors while avoiding the negative ones. According to research, a lack of sleep promotes forgetfulness, impulsivity, poor planning, and hyperactivity, all of which are indicators of ADHD. Massage may be given or received. You'll agree that getting a massage lowers tension. I don't think I need to reference any studies to persuade you of this. Massage has been shown in studies to have comparable benefits. According to a study conducted by academics at the University of Oxford and the ORYGEN Research Center (Mathews, 2021)

Massage has also been shown in other trials to alleviate pain, anxiety, and sadness. Strike a pact with your significant other to swap massages before bed, and you'll be astonished at the results. It doesn't take much to enjoy the many advantages of providing or getting a massage. About 10 or 15 minutes is plenty!

Alter your perspective on stress. We all know that stress is linked to poor mental and physical health and well-being, but what we don't realize is that our perception of it determines how damaging its consequences are. Stressing yourself out is what gets you into trouble.

Research undertaken by experts at the University of Denver discovered that if you can change your perspective on the things that stress you, you may protect yourself from inflicting significant harm to your health (Mathews, 2021). For example, you should not use an unpleasant circumstance as an excuse to skip a workout. Instead, consider it a chance to cultivate a virtue such as tolerance or patience. Difficult and terrible circumstances might make you stronger than you anticipated.

Go for a nature stroll at a park. If you read or listen to the tales of the world's most successful inventors and intellectuals, you will notice that they treasured lengthy walks in nature. Tchaikovsky, for example, was enthusiastic about his twice-daily walks because he believed they were critical to his health and creativity. Thomas Jefferson also went for daily walks around his Monticello residencee world's most successful inventors and intellectuals, you will notice that they treasured lengthy walks in nature. Tchaikovsky, for example, was enthusiastic about his twice-daily walks because he believed they were critical to his health and creativity. Thomas Jefferson also went for daily walks around his Monticello residence. According to studies, taking a 25-minute stroll in a park might decrease irritation and enhance mood (Mathews, 2021). Create more love. Remain closer than ever before. If you don't have much sex, increase the number of times you have sex in a week. Numerous studies have shown that having sex on a regular basis decreases stress, anxiety, and depression while also making you happier, more resilient, and improving your mood.

Listen to some classical music. According to research, classical music may emotionally engage you, sharpen your thinking, decrease blood pressure, alleviate physical discomfort and despair, and help you sleep better. Therefore, the next time you're worried, turn on some nice, peaceful, relaxing classical music.

Minimize the time you spend on your phones, computers, and TVs. According to studies, staring at screens for an extended period of time weakens your intellect. The more time you spend on computers and smartphones, the more agitated you get. According to research conducted by academics at the University of Gothenburg, the majority of symptoms linked with poor mental health are connected with excessive use of technology (Mathews, 2021). Individuals who use their computers and telephones without taking breaks are more likely to develop stress, sleep difficulties, and depression.

Use aromatherapy to your advantage. Just smelling lovely things might help you relax and lessen tension. Aromatherapy, or the scents of essential oils such as lavender, chamomile, geranium, and others, has been shown in studies to help decrease blood pressure, enhance sleep quality, and reduce anxiety. Incorporate it into your regular relaxing regimen by using a diffuser.

How to Discover Your Fitness Whys

To be successful on your fitness journey, set SMART objectives. Individuals who begin strength training activities with ambiguous, unachievable, or uninspired fitness objectives are the first to give up. They're also simple to detect. They will always have reasons and excuses to fall off the wagon. They will constantly moan about how circumstances and conditions have forced them to live a lazy and unhealthy lifestyle. If you want to succeed where others fail, avoid these attitudes and practices. That is why, in this part, we will undertake some soul-searching.

1. Describe your desired body type.

Whether you like it or not, the major reason most individuals exercise is to obtain a specific physical form and strength. And I'm sure this is the main reason you're here. Every physically fit person I know, including myself, is driven by how their body appears. I personally love and appreciate my health, but it would be a massive lie to say that it is the primary reason I engage in regular strength training.

So don't misinterpret me as egotistical. There are several physical advantages, but I don't see anything wrong with playing to our vanity if good looks make us feel more confident.

Thus, looking at your ideal physique today and imagining what you want to look like is one technique to determine your fitness objective. Take a photo of yourself with two or more of the physical traits you want and your ideal body form. Download these images to your phone, Google Drive, or another convenient location. This activity will give you the impression that you're working hard to get a true, ideal body form.

2. How does your ideal body feel?

This question allows you to delve into the "hidden" advantages of keeping physically active. The more fit and healthy you are, the higher your self-esteem, productivity, self-fulfillment, and self-confidence. Your emotions and alertness improve, and you also have more energy, clearer thinking, fewer pains, and better sleep. Therefore, spend a few minutes envisioning what these sensations might be like for you and then write them down in your diary as physical affirmations. Make a list of positive phrases that describe how you want to be. For those who are unfamiliar with affirmations, this is what I meant. "I'm full of vigor and vitality," or "my self-esteem is always high," are two examples.

3. Your physical fitness Why does it change as you change?

If you keep on track, fitness can be an incredible trip. Exercise will most likely cause changes in your physical appearance as well as your willpower, confidence, health, strength, and motivation. Your fitness objectives will vary as a result of these modifications. You must rewrite the new objectives in the same way that you did the old ones. Remember that your objectives are a big part of why you got this far, so don't lose sight of them. Instead, go back to where you began and set new objectives to help you accomplish something you never thought possible at the start.

Monitoring Your Progress

You can only know where you're going if you can quantify and communicate your progress in actual figures. Many individuals fail to meet their fitness objectives because they lack a regular, objective means to track their progress.

How carefully you monitor your progress will determine much of your future success or failure. We monitor improvement using three components: body composition, food, and activity. But, for the purposes of this book, we will simply need to monitor our body composition and exercise. Let us investigate more.

Monitoring Your Body Composition

Body composition analysis is essential for any fitness quest. It is important to note that even if you do everything correctly throughout your training, it may take longer than expected to see improvements in your physical appearance. This might cause you to lose hope and give up.

Nevertheless, if you learn how to correctly monitor your body composition, you can avoid this issue. With effective body composition tracking, you can always know precisely what is or isn't occurring with your body, allowing you to make modifications accordingly. The steps for monitoring your body composition are as follows:

1. Weigh yourself every day and compute weekly averages. Your weight fluctuates on a daily basis due to fluid retention, glycogen levels, and bowel movements. It is sometimes up and sometimes down. As a result, experiencing frequent ups and downs is common. That is why it is critical to weigh oneself every day and compute your weekly average. You will be able to concentrate on the ultimate outcomes rather than being too concerned and disturbed by daily variations, which may cause undue irritation and confusion. If your average weight rises, you are gaining weight, and if it falls, you are losing weight. That's all there is to it.

Here's how it's done:

Weigh yourself naked after you've used the restroom and before you drink or take anything in the morning.
Add together the daily weigh-ins and divide by seven to obtain the daily average weight after seven days.
Make a note of your averages in your notepad app, Google Sheets, or someplace else you can readily retrieve them.
2. Measure your body once a week. Even with meticulous recording, your weight cannot tell you how your body evolves. Weight monitoring does not reveal what you're gaining or losing—is it muscle or fat? If you are new to strength training and want to lose fat, you may expect to increase muscle while losing fat. This implies that your scale's numbers may not vary as much as you think. That is why, in addition to your weight, it is critical to record at least one body measurement per week. You should keep an eye on your waist circumference. Your waist circumference is a good predictor of fat reduction or growth. It may help you determine if you're gaining or losing fat. As a result, in addition to calculating your daily average

body weight, measure the diameter of your waist at the conclusion of each week and track it over time.

Here's how to do it correctly:
Put a tape measure around your naked stomach, just at your navel. Check that the tape measure is not slanted and is parallel to the floor. Hug your body slightly without compressing the skin. Breathe out while you take the measurements. Make sure you don't flex or suck your stomach in.

To guarantee that your measurements are consistent, take the measurement in the same location each time.

3. Take weekly progress photos. The majority of us are more interested in what we see in the mirror than with statistics. That is why some individuals prefer photographs over measurements. It is critical to take your "before" shots there, even if you don't like your look at the moment. These images will make you adore how your body will change over the coming weeks and months. And you'll probably be surprised at how much your body has improved over time. Take weekly progress shots as well as weekly measurements to watch how the change develops.

Keeping Track of Your Workout

Exercise and body composition monitoring are equally crucial. Only by tracking your strength training workouts can you assure that you are gradually overloading your muscles over time. These are some techniques for keeping track of your exercise:

Maintain an exercise diary. Journaling is one of the most basic and efficient methods to keep track of your exercise progress. You may note the amount of weight you lifted in prior workouts by keeping a workout diary. This indicates whether or not you are growing stronger. Our bodies quickly adapt to whatever activities we do on a regular basis.

As a result, if we continue to lift the same weights and execute the same repetitions, our bodies will no longer respond to change. This implies that your muscles will not develop or get stronger. This is the error that the majority of us make. A fitness diary may help with this. It assists you in keeping your muscles challenged at all times. Make use of a pen and paper. This tracking practice is just as straightforward as it sounds. It is also the least expensive method of planning and monitoring your exercises. All you need is a book and a pen to write down all of the exercises, the number of sets and repetitions you will do, the weights you will lift, and so on. Make good use of your phone. You may use any app or particular application for notes. When I don't perform strength training sessions, I prefer to use Google Calendar to designate days for strength workouts and days for other physical activity, like going for a walk. The calendar allows me to keep track of my activities and ensure that I get adequate relaxation in between sessions. You may also make comments in calendar events for workouts if you need assistance monitoring your weights and repetitions, but I don't. For me, having a photo of my workout on my phone is sufficient to ensure that I did not skip any exercises.

Motivating Yourself to Workout

Knowing why we exercise and establishing wise objectives, being prepared, having discipline and dedication, and other factors all contribute to a regular exercise regimen. Yet there is one that is crucial and, at times, elusive: motivation. Your mental state is an essential component of any long-term muscular and strength-building program. Of course, you need the weights, repetitions, sets, and rest in between to build lean muscle mass, but your mental state will influence whether or not you start and stick with it.

Numerous factors might reduce your enthusiasm for exercise, particularly if you have to do it from home. The good news is that there are various strategies to overcome any barriers to exercise and stay motivated. Here are a few alternatives to think about:

Establish objectives. Take some time to set your objectives before beginning your strength training regimen. Establish a few achievable short- and long-term objectives that take into consideration your current situation and priorities. Determine what you want to accomplish and how you will carry out your strategy.

Prepare for the workout. Know what exercise you'll perform, how long it'll take, and what you'll need to complete it. Make sure you have everything you need for each workout.

Begin gently. If you haven't been exercising, don't start a high-intensity fitness regimen right away. Start small and gradually progress. Begin by dividing your exercises into 10-minute chunks twice a day, with as few as 3 repeats of 2 sets in each activity. If you have continuous cardiac issues or are afraid of falling, start with simple chair exercises. This will allow you to gradually improve your fitness and confidence.

Reward yourself for working out. Don't forget to praise yourself for every exercise you do, no matter how little. For example, if you worked out for 30 minutes in the morning, you might spend an hour listening to music, watching a movie, or reading a book. You might also set aside money each month for a larger incentive, such as a safari. Knowing you'll receive a reward after you work out is terrific motivation.

Maintain a record of your workout progress. Assessing and appreciating your accomplishments is the most effective approach to remaining motivated to exercise. Track all of your daily workouts, monitor your weekly and monthly progress to determine whether you've improved, and then adjust your exercise plan depending on your results.

Discover methods to make it more pleasurable. Find something innovative that will help you stick to your training program. Note that although most individuals dislike strength training, there are benefits to it. You may begin by lifting your children while you play with them, walking your dog, and so on. Just do something you like while keeping up with the pace.

Make fitness a social event. Consider exercising with others if you want to achieve your fitness goals. When done with others, activities are usually more fun. Exercise alone might demotivate you and cause you to quiters if you want to achieve your fitness goals. When done with others, activities are usually more fun. Exercise alone might demotivate you and cause you to quit. If at all feasible, have a workout companion or someone you can rely on for accountability. You may take a dancing class, utilize family gatherings to undertake outdoor activities, participate in a charity run, or play team sports with your children.

Strength training becomes easy once you have started. Establishing a habit of working out on a regular basis is more important in attaining your fitness objectives and obtaining the greatest advantages from strength training, even as you get older. Motivation is one of our most difficult challenges on our path. But, rather than just losing desire, it is critical to consider what you would benefit from exercising. Those who exercise, like myself, make every effort to find reasons to do so. They understand that exercise improves one's quality of life. Hence, if you're lacking motivation to exercise, consider the advantages.

Important Takeaways

Strength training is good at any age, but it is especially advantageous for those over the age of 40.

You'll get the most benefits from exercise if you do it regularly and with discipline and self-control. As a result, you must do all you can to improve it.

If you want to get the most out of exercise and reach your full health and fitness potential, you need to be mentally motivated and ready for the road ahead.

People who start strength training but don't have clear, attainable, or inspiring fitness goals are the first to quit. Don't be one of them; instead, discover the "smart" fitness whys.

Why is Cardio Exercise a Waste of Time?

Have you ever gone to the gym a few times per week without seeing any results?You may be wondering why this entire workout isn't working. I've seen folks who go to the gym yet have no influence on their body. Many individuals put in long hours of cardio in the hopes of seeing greater results, only to be let down. I'd hate for you to go through the same thing. Strength training is the key to decreasing body fat and developing muscle.

During strength training, the metabolism causes the lean muscle tissue to burn calories throughout the exercise and throughout the day. Isn't it incredible? Strength training helps to enhance posture and the body. Also, when you burn calories, it improves your cardio and allows you to do other tasks more effectively.

While most individuals favor aerobic workouts like running, swimming, or bicycling, several studies show that they are ineffective for reducing weight and increasing muscle. According to research, some people who engage in cardiovascular activity wind up being heavier than they began. Cardio may not always provide noticeable outcomes. Replacing the expended calories in your body is usually relatively simple.

For instance, if a man ran vigorously for 30 minutes, he would likely burn approximately 300 calories (but only up to 200 calories with low-impact cardio).Surprisingly, you can get the same number of calories from a bagel, a doughnut, a burger, or two cans of cola.So, which is simpler? Running on the treadmill for 30 minutes or foregoing the bagel? Additionally, whether we exercise or not, our bodies burn around 100 calories each hour, which should be subtracted from the "calories burned" shown on the treadmill's screen.

It is even more vital to be mindful of your diet when exercising. Maintain healthy eating habits that complement your fitness routine. Cardiovascular workouts do not burn as many calories as we would like to lose weight. It will also not help you acquire strength or get in shape.

Cardio, in addition to burning fewer calories than necessary, causes your body to adapt to calorie-reduction routines. According to scientists, when your body is in a calorie deficit, the efficiency of energy production falls, and as you workout, the amount of energy needed to accomplish the same activities decreases. As a consequence, even if you execute the same workouts you began with under the same circumstances, you will not burn as many calories as you thought. In this instance, you are likely to overeat, putting a halt to your weight reduction attempts. When this occurs, the only option is to do more and more exercise to speed up the loss of energy levels. Yet, it may result in muscle loss and a decrease in metabolic rate in the body. Clearly, cardiovascular activities may not be the best strategy to obtain the physique you want.

You want to be strong, muscular, and athletic if you're like most men. This is often the reason we begin to workout with weights. Cardio cannot provide the same outcomes. Consider athletes or those who run often but do not strength train; the majority of them are constantly slim with no visible muscles, and others may have a skinny-fat body composition. Look at those people who never run but constantly undertake weightlifting exercises; the majority of them have well-defined muscle mass, buffed chests and arms, and robust, huge bodies. So, what body type do you prefer? You have an option.

If you're like most women, you desire a toned figure with a well-formed stomach that gives you the confidence to flaunt about. To be honest, exercise will never give you this kind of body form. Strength training workouts will be required. Most women, however, avoid weightlifting owing to the popular misconception that it makes you bulky. Yet the truth is that testosterone, or the absence thereof, is one of the key reasons why women don't bulk up from weightlifting. Testosterone is a natural anabolic steroid that promotes muscular development. In addition, women have one-seventh the quantity of testosterone as men. If you've ever seen a fat lady, chances are she's on steroids.

So why am I so adamant about strength training?

Strength training does not require you to spend all day lifting weights; you may get big effects by doing it for 30 minutes twice a week. Your muscles will improve as you continue strength exercises. You may acquire the strength to lift additional weight after each workout.
Your body adjusts to burning extra fat while you workout. Strength training increases your body's metabolic rate, allowing you to burn calories for a longer period of time after working out. Numerous studies have indicated that your body loses roughly 129 calories per day for every 3 pounds of lean muscle.

Strength training also helps you cope with certain muscles at work. This minimizes the chance of having reduced bone mass, decreased mobility, impaired coordination, imbalance, and inflexibility. Moreover, strength training forces your muscles to get stronger, resulting in speedy results. This boosts your body image and, hence, your self-confidence. Lifting weights helps build muscle by producing resistance. The tissues degrade fast, causing the body to clean them up and mend them. Muscles develop and get stronger throughout this process. As a result, you should routinely press your muscles to the point of development and train them to fatigue; nevertheless, as a novice, you may start with a simple, basic plan that you level up over time.

Strength training, as opposed to aerobics, strengthens the region surrounding the joints. Your range of motion and capacity to undertake greater weight lifting grow as your joints get stronger. When you lift weights correctly, the core parts of our joints boost the flow of your action. As a result, when you exercise, your body learns to withstand these motions, lowering the chances of damage throughout the workout. You will see and feel the effects of added weight training workouts as you train yourself. Isn't that what you're after?

Strength training may be done at home or at the gym. Body weight is one of the most prevalent types of strength training. This may be done with very little or no equipment. Pushups, pullups, planks, lunges, and squats are a few examples.

Bands of resistance. This is a low-cost way of creating resistance when one stretches using lightweight bands. There are several varieties of resistance bands available at sporting goods stores. Another kind of strength training that uses traditional training materials is free weights. Dumbbells and kettlebells are excellent options to explore. If you don't have access to free weight at home, you may substitute a gallon of water or sand, or you can improvise with old auto components.

Machines for lifting weights They are available at fitness establishments. You may also buy one to use at home. Suspension training involves suspending a portion of your body. Suspend your legs when completing push-ups or planks, for example.

Overall, moving your body is preferable to being absolutely sedentary. If the prospect of exercising every day frustrates you, make an attempt to move your body. Don't simply sit on the sofa. Even five minutes of walking may have an impact. I want you to let go of the notion that jogging must cover a certain number of miles in order to be deemed an activity. From your brain to your joints, performing basic and modest motions may vastly enhance your health and have a huge influence on achieving a physically fit physique.

As a result, I recommend that you get moving and avoid becoming idle. Search out an activity that you like and commit to performing it every day. For example, if you like walking, remind yourself to walk for 30 minutes every day. Walking, swimming, golfing, or any other low-intensity activity that you have the discipline to perform regularly can provide excellent benefits.

According to research, one of the primary reasons humans have brains is to make flexible and complicated motions. Our daily activities are carried out through movement. The most crucial thing for you to grasp is that bodily mobility aids in the maintenance of excellent health. Many individuals have a negative attitude about the term "exercise," particularly when it comes to weightlifting or strength training. People link it with worry and responsibility. You now realize that strength training is beneficial to your health after reading this book—consider exercising to be simply moving. It should never seem too complicated.

Thus, if working out gives you a bad sensation, attempt to adjust your mindset. Nevertheless, you must keep your body moving to remain physically active. Walking about while chatting on the phone is one of the simplest ways to achieve this, particularly if the conversation is with someone you speak to often. You may also just go around your home picking up dirt or lost belongings, or go to a nearby park and wander around. All of these moves add up. They have a big impact on your physical and emotional well-being. The good news is that you can test them out in the comfort of your own home without even changing into your gym clothes. Some activities to exercise your body include decluttering and organizing your garage or basement. You will be lugging heavy goods from one location to another, bending and crouching to pick things up, and so forth.

Walking on foot to the store

In the winter, digging snow; in the summer, swimming in a lake or river Gardening is also a fantastic kind of exercise. Walking, squatting, moving your hands, pushing, and pulling are all part of it. All of them are good methods to get your body moving. Take advantage of the great outdoors. You can walk your dog, ride your bike, hike, or jog. Moving your body outdoors exposes you to nature, which improves your mental wellness.

Moving your body is typically beneficial. Thus, if working out seems like a chore, try these basic routines that integrate movement into your everyday life and make you feel wonderful. Hence, depending on your tastes, you may adjust your workout regimen. You may achieve your strenuous objectives a lot more easily without compromising your fun.

Strength training is important to keep your body active, balanced, strong, healthy, and in great shape because it helps you burn more fat and keep your muscles in less time than cardio. Now that we've established that, let's look at everything you'll need for your strength training activity in the next chapter. So first, what's the bottom line here?

Important Takeaways

You don't need cardio to have the strong, healthy, and attractive physique you want, but you do need strength training. Women, no matter how much weight they lift, can never bulk up. Their hormones do not allow for this. Yet, for guys, sure! Their hormones make it possible.

Moving your body is quite beneficial. Don't simply sit on the sofa. If you can't start strength training right away, start with easy motions. It is more vital to be careful of your diet than to concentrate heavily on cardiac workouts.

Will You Need a Lot of Workout Equipment?

You should now see why it is critical to strength train as you reach middle age and even beyond. I cannot emphasize enough how important strength training is for getting in shape and building bodily strength. The key concern today is whether or not you need a lot of equipment to do the workouts. And if you do need them, what should you choose?

If you're like me and have been doing strength training activities to stay healthy, you'll agree that the majority of these workouts require very little equipment. And if you're new to strength training, disregard everything you've heard about it and start here. Strength training does not require the use of expensive or specialized weightlifting equipment or gym-style machinery.

If your money is limited, you may even improvise by utilizing furniture or other objects from your home to do the exercises. To get the most out of your fitness program, though, it is important to invest in at least one or two pieces of equipment. And free weights are an excellent option!

Bodyweight exercises may also be used, but they require certain equipment, such as pull-up bars and parallel bars, which might be difficult to install and use at home. Yet, free weights are simpler and easier to use. As a result, I feel they are the best choice for everyone interested in weightlifting.

Dumbbells, kettlebells, weight plates, weight sets, and other weight training equipment are examples of free weights. Utilizing free weights is a great approach to shedding fat and improving power and muscle. The ability of free weights to completely activate all of the muscles in the body makes them an excellent and efficient workout tool for strength and muscular gain. There are several advantages to utilizing free weights in your strength training routine. This implies that if you're serious about getting in shape and growing muscle, you should invest in a kettlebell or dumbbell. These are some of the benefits of using free weights:

They serve a purpose. Outside of the gym, regular exercise should enhance your performance. This is what we call functional fitness or exercise, and it requires free weights. Free weights provide a more natural motion that corresponds to your body's normal, functioning activity. Unlike machines, which normally limit you to a single plane of motion, Even simple free weight exercises like the standing dumbbell biceps curl employ the hands in the same way as you would in everyday chores like carrying groceries or shopping bags. It is particularly crucial as you get older to keep your natural, complete range of motion.

They help you become stronger. The way your body responds to free weights differs from how it responds to machines. Squatting with free weights versus squatting with a machine, for example, has quite distinct effects on your muscles. Squatting with free weights increases muscular activation and hormone reactions. When you workout, the hormones help your muscles develop and heal (Fetters, 2019).

They are transportable. Can you bring resistance machines with you when you travel? Or will they fit in your closet? Very likely not. But what about a lightweight dumbbell? It is entirely feasible. Consider investing in free weights if you want to save money and space. They help you maintain your equilibrium. Unlike machines, which require you to move the weight in just one plane of motion, free weights need your muscles to balance the weight in all planes. This causes your muscles to cooperate, which improves balance, coordination, and muscular development.

They have more adaptability. There are no restrictions on free weights. You may execute a number of exercises that engage all of your muscles in various ways to strengthen them with only a basic pair of kettlebells or dumbbells and a few square feet of vacant space. Apart from supporting muscular development, diversified exercise may make your exercises more enjoyable, inspiring you to stick to your routine.

Free weights are more effective. Unlike machines that force you to push or pull in one direction, free weights integrate stabilizing muscles that allow you to perform the action. You must also keep the weights and yourself from swaying. This increases the effectiveness of free weights in terms of general physical strength and power improvements.

They lower your chance of harm. Lifting free weights helps to correct muscular imbalances and thereby avoid injuries. Since free weights continuously test your balance while exercising, they require you to engage and build your stabilizing muscles, producing stability to help support your body and joints. Moreover, free weights might be of varying weights. Dumbbells and kettlebells of various weights are commonly available. This allows you to adjust the weights to a size that you can lift comfortably and safely. They expend more calories. Not only can free weights increase your stability, but they also guarantee that your complete body executes complex motions. More calories are burned when you exercise more muscles. For example, if you do kettlebell goblet squats, you train your legs, core, arms, and shoulders, which improves the quantity of calories expended when compared to a workout that isolates a particular muscle, such as calf raises.

They are more affordable. Free weights are inexpensive. If you are serious about building a strong, attractive, and healthy physique, you can buy at least a dumbbell or kettlebell. A little investment is well worth the return.

Strength training on gym equipment might be scary. As a result, when it comes to designing a healthy and safe strength training program, free weights are the better choice. If you investigate the great strength athletes and bodybuilders, you will find that they employed free weights in their strength training to reach their goals. Hence, using free weights in strength training is a solid approach to getting the results you want from your session. Let's take a deeper look at the kettlebells and dumbbells, two of the most popular, efficient, and effective free weights used in strength training.

Kettlebell Exercise

A kettlebell is a cast-iron ball with a top handle. Kettlebells are available in a variety of weights and can help you burn up to 400 calories in 20 minutes (Smith, 2020). Squats, lunges, shoulder presses, hinges, and lifts can all be done with a kettlebell. As you work out with a kettlebell, your heart rate increases slightly, burning almost 20 calories per minute.

Kettlebells improve flexibility since you may incorporate various techniques into your training. Kettlebell exercises are often high-intensity because they include fast-paced cardio and strength training techniques. It primarily targets the core, arms, legs, shoulders, and back.

Dumbbells are short bars with weights at one end that may be fixed or movable to produce a range of weights. All you have to do is change the settings to suit your demands and the progress of the activity. Adjustable dumbbells are ideal for households with more than one individual who needs to exercise.

Dumbells also work well for isolated workouts. If you want to train certain muscles, such as your biceps, bicep curls with a dumbbell are the best option.

Benefits of Kettlebells and Dumbbells

They take up very little storage space. You may use them to exercise and then stow them in the corner of the room to free up space for other activities.

They are multipurpose. They are inexpensive compared to other gym equipment, making them affordable. They promote coordination and stability of muscles and joints. They increase the flexibility of your muscles and joints, providing you with functional strength. They build your cardiovascular endurance to a high level. Kettlebell workouts can burn up to 20 calories per minute. They help improve your body's coordination and mental

They allow you to add weight in little increments rather than large bricks at a time. Since most dumbbells are adjustable, you may gradually increase the amount of weight you're lifting. This allows you to strengthen your muscles properly.

All you need to know about free weights

Kettlebells and dumbbells range in price from $10 to $100, depending on weight. The heavier the kettlebell, the higher the price.

Signing up for a class to learn the fundamentals of kettlebell and dumbbell exercises is recommended, particularly if you are a novice. You will choose the proper weight for you as you learn more about it.
Depending on your preferences, you may practice kettlebell or dumbbell training indoors or outside the home. You might also enroll in a gym class that includes a kettlebell or dumbbell exercise. Which is superior? Dumbbells or kettlebells?

Any of these fantastic gadgets may be used to exercise all of your muscles without the need for a gym membership. None of them is clearly better than the other. A kettlebell may be used for every activity that a dumbbell can be used for. But I love kettlebells because they add excitement and enjoyment to my training. So, do you want to amp up your workout? Kettlebells are your best bet. They assist in burning more calories in a shorter period of time. A kettlebell workout may include both strength training and aerobic activities, depending on the regimen you follow. As a result, before you begin, you should contact a health professional. Of course, achieving optimal outcomes with a kettlebell exercise begins with your mental state.

Have a prepared attitude and handle the exercise with respect. This means you must be diligent enough not to miss any workouts. It is also a good idea to assess what works best for you. Certain kettlebells may be too heavy for you, resulting in shoulder, back, or neck issues. As a result, be certain that you are thoroughly informed of all facts and how to use the kettlebells by an expert trainer, who will advise you to prevent any danger of injury throughout the workout. If you've already exercised, using a kettlebell can help you burn more calories in less time. Also, your muscles and stamina will grow considerably quicker than previously.

The advantage of kettlebells is that they may be used for both high- and low-intensity workouts. You may lift them as hard as you want, or you can use them for gentler exercises if sweating isn't your thing. Kettlebells are my absolute favorites, and I always prefer them. That is why I will demonstrate how to complete the workouts in our program using a kettlebell. This does not imply that you must execute the exercises with a kettlebell. You are free to utilize a dumbbell or another free weight if you have one.

What if you have a medical problem? Is it possible to utilize free weights?
In such a circumstance, a doctor's advice is required. As a result, if your doctor approves of the use of free weights in your workout

program, you are free to do so. For example, if you have diabetes and your doctor allows you to use free weights, you will develop muscle and reduce fat more quickly. As a consequence, your blood sugar level will drop. Working out with free weights may also help lower blood pressure and cholesterol levels. But if you have a cardiac condition, you should see your doctor before doing any free-weight exercise.

Kettlebells, being a high-impact workout, put pressure on your hip, back, shoulder, knee, and neck muscles. Hence, if you have problems like arthritis that cause knee or back discomfort, you should choose less dangerous strength training regimens like body weight. As a result, I've included alternate workouts that you may perform without any equipment in my routine.

If you have any additional health issues, get the advice of an expert trainer to determine the best training regimen for you.

Several trainers and scientists believe that using free weights in strength training is the most effective approach to building your muscles, burning more calories, enhancing your whole-body flexibility, and becoming better at everything you do (Fetters, 2019). Nevertheless, in order to get the full advantages of free weight training, you must learn how to apply force when you lift them. It is easier to prevent injuries when you practice utilizing the right abilities. Do you want to know how?

Don't worry; I'll go over this in a future chapter. We will master proper form for lifting some of the most efficient and effective free weights. For every core exercise, we will also offer a bodyweight variation. But I feel that using weights, particularly kettlebells, is the most effective way to do core exercises. The best part about utilizing free weights is that you can workout anywhere, including outdoors, in gyms, and in your own home. To prevent having restricted strength with machines, utilize free weights for a decent exercise.

Important Takeaways

Strength training routines do not need a lot of equipment. A kettlebell or dumbbells will assist you in doing the majority of strength training routines and reaping all of the benefits.

A single kettlebell can activate all the muscles in the body. The benefit of free weights like kettlebells and dumbbells is that they are inexpensive and customizable. You can acquire one for between $10 and $100. As you feel the desire to lift additional weight, you may use various weights to advance.

Practice the Moves

In this chapter, I will introduce the six best compound exercises for increasing overall muscle mass and strength and getting into your desired shape in no time. A compound exercise involves multiple joints and trains multiple muscles at the same time, allowing you to lift heavier weights and increase growth hormone and testosterone levels. This means more time efficiency, faster muscle growth, and a slew of other advantages.

When describing each move, I will first introduce and focus on my recommended exercise, followed by alternative variations. Each exercise in this section meets the program's requirements. I conducted extensive research to ensure that I am providing you with a group of exercises that will work in tandem to provide maximum results with minimal effort.

These exercises are designed to make you better, not worse. And to do so, you must carry them out correctly. So, begin slowly, carefully follow all instructions, and watch the results! Let's get started!

Squats
Squats are the best exercise for leg development and may be the best overall exercise to perform if you want to strengthen your body. This is the king of all exercises. Squatting is something we were born to do, and everyone on the planet has done it. It is one of the first movements that children learn.

Before they can walk upright, babies must first perform squats. Unfortunately, we no longer embrace it as we get older. We regard it as a significant developmental milestone for children. And as we get older, we become accustomed to sitting and forget that we are supposed to be able to squat effortlessly. As a result, we lose the flexibility, strength, and balance required to squat without falling over. The good news is that we can still do something about it—squatting exercises.

When we mention squats as an exercise, most people think of the barbell back squat. Although this is the most well-known variation of squats, it is not the only one, nor is it the one I recommend. Back squats with a barbell require a lot of energy, a trainer (if you're new to it), a squat rack, and the barbell with weights itself. You can't have all of these at home. That's why I recommend simple variations that you can do from anywhere, like this one: the goblet kettlebell squat.

The goblet kettlebell squat
This is one of the most effective squat variations you can do. It is also one of the simplest full-body exercises to perform. It works your quads, glutes, calves, and core. Because you engage your hands by holding the weight, it also works your biceps, improving your arm and grip strength.

Its advantages
The counterbalance makes it simpler and easier to perform the goblet squat safely and correctly. It also has a shorter learning curve, making it an excellent teaching tool for learning how to perform.

Begin by standing upright and holding a kettlebell in front of your chest with both hands on the sides of its handle. Your shoulders should be drawn back and downward, and your elbows should be tucked in closer to the kettlebell. Keep your forearms as vertical as possible. Your feet should be slightly wider than your shoulders. Take a deep breath and tighten your core. Maintain a straight back and a straight chest, hinge at the hips, and sit back as if on an invisible chair. Continue lowering yourself as far as you can while keeping your head, chest, and back straight.

As you descend, spread your knees. You should be able to feel the majority of your weight distributed between your heel and midfoot. Don't round your lower back. If you feel your lower back starting to round, stop and come back up.

Do not lean forward or struggle to keep the bell upright. Your torso should remain vertical; don't bend or twist either side. Exhale as you stand back up. Put equal weight on both legs, making sure your heels stay planted on the floor at all times. To maintain an upright posture throughout the movement, your knees, hips, and back should all move at the same rate.

Avoiding common form errors

Leaning forward. The kettlebell goblet squat, like any other squat variation, requires you to keep your chest up at all times when performing this move. This assists in keeping your center of gravity on your feet.

Leaning back. This helps keep your lats tight throughout the movement, allowing your body to stay balanced and stable. To do this, imagine someone is tickling you from behind and draw your elbows in towards your sides.

I'm wobbling. Make sure to begin each rep with your entire torso engaged. This makes it more stable, resulting in a more smooth and controlled movement. Concentrate on tightening and tensing your lower back, abs, and glutes.

You can also perform this move with a dumbbell or resistance band. If you are a beginner or have physical limitations that may make this movement pattern difficult, try bodyweight squats or bodyweight squats with a TRX belt, chair or box squats, or even shallow knee bends.

The Hinge

The hinge is one of the most effective and efficient workouts for general health and well-being. Regrettably, it is the most ignored. Most of us spend a lot of time sitting. This stresses your back and spine, resulting in back discomfort. In addition, as we age, most individuals have back and joint discomfort. Fortunately, if not avoided, these aches may be addressed. The best therapy strategy is to do hinge exercises. Here are some easy hinge exercises:

The kettlebell swing

Kettlebells are fantastic, and I feel that the kettlebell swing is the finest alternative for hinge movements! Pavel Tsatsouline, the inventor of kettlebell training in the United States and author of multiple books, discovered that kettlebell swing has various advantages, including increasing the number of repetitions you can accomplish in a pull-up exercise and improving strength in others. Pavel describes a minimalistic workout in one of his books that consists of just two movements, one of which is swinging. This indicates how effective this workout is. The kettlebell swing is a full-body reaction exercise, according to most specialists. It offers several advantages for your muscles and overall health. Here's how to get started and get the most out of this practice.

Put up a kettlebell in front of your feet.

Stand tall with your feet slightly wider than shoulder width apart and your toes pointing slightly outward. To activate your abs, bend your knees slightly, roll your shoulders back, and draw in your navel.
Thrust your hips back and tilt your body forward to reach your hand for the kettlebell's grip. While you do this, make sure your back is absolutely straight and you're not crouching.

Breathe deeply as you securely grip the handle of the kettlebell with both hands, shoulders back. This helps with swing control. Remember to keep your core engaged throughout the workout. To begin the swing, hike the kettlebell back between your legs until it is stretched behind your back. When you reach your feet, exhale.

Do not extend your hips beyond your shoulders. Let the bell swing forward as far as it naturally can.

Breathe in and swing the kettlebell back to the floor through your legs at a calm and controlled pace, then exhale and repeat.

Avoiding Common Form Errors

When you swing, squat. Recall that the kettle swing is a hinge action, not a squat. This implies that instead of bending at the knee, you should force your hips back whenever you execute a downward swing. The shins should remain mainly vertical. Rounding your back. A rounded or drooping upper body indicates that your core and shoulder stabilizers are not correctly engaged, which may cause lower back discomfort or strain. To prevent this, keep your spine and back as straight as possible.

Raising using the arms and shoulders Most individuals blame their shoulders and arms for the kettlebell's forward movement. The kettlebell should be moved by your hips rather than your arms. Your arms should only work to hold the bell, not to hoist it. Maintain a relaxed yet solid posture with your shoulders and upper back. To swing the weight, try to depend as much as possible on the momentum of your hip extension.

Alternate hinge exercises

If you are a beginner or have physical restrictions that may make this exercise difficult, consider more basic hinge variants like the kettlebell deadlift or bodyweight alternatives like the hip raise and standing back extensions.

The kettlebell deadlift

Standing erect with a kettlebell between your feet, hinge at your hips backward while keeping your back straight, bend your knees while maintaining a straight back with your chest elevated, and hold the kettlebell handles with both hands and push into the ground to rise up. Lift the kettlebell slightly above your knees, maintaining your arms straight. Make sure your glutes are firm and you're not leaning back.

This counts as one rep.

Warm-ups are usually recommended to minimize muscle injuries. If you are new to this exercise, begin with a lightweight kettlebell. Avoid hunching at your lower back. That might cause a major back injury. Always hinge at the hips.

The Advantages of Kettlebell Deadlift

It engages several muscles in your body, including the quadriceps, hamstrings, glutes, forearms, core, and so on. It improves your posture. It sculpts your whole core and body. The dynamic movements of the kettlebell increase muscular connection and mental attention, and it is quite safe. Kettlebells place significantly less strain on your spine than other standard equipment like barbells, and they build grip strength.

Standing-Back-Extension

Standing tall with your feet together, spin your hip joint to bend forward.
Extend your hands, keeping your knees straight, to bring your fingers in line with the tips of your toes.

Check that your knees are not locked. You may avoid this by microbending them.

Maintain maximum quadriceps engagement and straight legs without hyperextending.

Let your head dangle and attempt to shift your weight to the balls of your feet.

Pause for a few seconds.

To return to the beginning posture, inhale and engage your abdominal muscles as you gently rise.
Repeat as many times as you can.
Body Form Mistakes to Avoid
Rounding your upper back
Rolling your shoulders forward, locking your knees, and rounding your lower back

Hip raise

Begin by lying on your back on the floor with your knees bent, feet flat on the floor, and shins upright.

For stability, place your hands on the floor at your sides, palms facing up.

Raise your hips off the floor by pressing your feet into the ground and using your glutes and back muscles.

Continue to raise your hips forward while pressing down with your heels until they connect with your shoulders and knees. Maintain that position for 2 seconds.

To return to the beginning posture, slowly lower your hips to the floor in a controlled move.

3. The push-up

The push-up is one of the most fundamental bodyweight exercises that may help you improve your upper-body strength, muscular mass, and pressing ability. It focuses on the muscles of the chest, arms, and shoulders. It also strengthens your core and helps you create stabilizer muscles throughout your whole body. Push-ups have the advantage of not requiring any equipment. You may do them from anywhere at any time.

These are simple to learn and practice. They are basic upper body hypertrophy exercises to strengthen the chest, triceps, and anterior shoulder. You may utilize them to acquire the physical control and strength required for more advanced exercises.

Start in a high plank stance with your back straight. Hands should be somewhat wider than shoulder width apart, with palms flat, fingers splayed, and facing forward. Maintain your abdominals firm, buttocks compressed, and back flat. Engage your core and glutes. Your legs should be completely stretched behind you, with your feet and thighs aggressively squeezed together. Maintain a neutral head position to keep your whole body straight.

Pull your shoulder blades together to produce tension in your upper back. This improves your stability as you lower yourself. Bend your elbows and lower your body until your chest hits the floor. Your head and shoulders should not sag forward toward the floor. Make sure your thighs, hips, and chest all make contact with the floor at the same moment. Your whole body should be in a straight line. Gaze at a point a foot or two ahead of you to help maintain a neutral neck. Keep your elbows tucked in and parallel to your body. As you contact the floor, push through your hands and drive yourself away and upwards to return to the beginning position.

While completing push-ups, keep your body form in mind. Never, ever round your back. Maintain a straight back throughout the movement; focus on using your muscles even during the lowering phase; and always keep your abdomen and buttocks firm to stabilize your core during push-ups.

Press your weight through your whole hand, including the fingers. This helps reduce wrist strain. Remember to breathe throughout the motions.
Quit the instant you recognize your privacy is being compromised.

Alternate push workouts

If you are a novice or have physical restrictions that may make this action difficult, consider gentler varieties such as knee push-ups, wall push-ups, and slope push-ups. Therefore, as you grow, if you feel like you need something more difficult to test your muscular power, try to avoid doing push-ups.

Knee push-ups

Knee push-ups are performed in the same manner as push-ups, except on your knees.

Begin by kneeling on the floor.

Stretch your arms on the floor in front of you. Hands should be shoulder-width apart, palms flat, fingers wide, and pointing forward. Hold your abs firm as you bend your elbows and lower your body until your chest reaches the floor.

Return to the beginning posture by pushing through your hands and pressing your torso away and upward. The movement should be moderate and steady. Don't rush your body.

Complete 10–15 repetitions.

Incline push-ups

A strong box, bench, or table is required for this.

Standing facing the box, bench, or table, bend down and put both hands on the edges of each side of the box. Make sure your hands are somewhat wider than shoulder width apart.

Maintain your arms straight (don't lock your elbows) and position your feet to ensure your torso is absolutely straight. (Your head should be in line with your spine.) Next, bend your elbows to help you progressively lower your chest toward the edge of the box while you breathe in. Maintain a straight and firm body as you do this action.

Exhale as you push yourself up by straightening your arms until your elbows are completely stretched but not locked.

Formal blunders to avoid

Putting your hands out too far This decreases the range of motion of the workouts, lowering their overall efficacy.

Bad alignment. Your whole body should be straight. Slump, droop, or bend your hips or knees. Your upper and lower bodies should be in perfect alignment.

Shorter range of motion. With each rep, go through your whole range of motion, from straight arms to completely bent arms. If you're a newbie and can't accomplish the whole range, stick to wall push-ups.

Push-ups on a Wall

Standing a few feet away from a wall, lean in slightly and rest your hands on the wall at chest level, somewhat wider than shoulder width.
Inhale as you slowly and carefully bend your elbows and lower your body toward the wall. Pull your abs in and keep a straight back as you do this action.

Move until your elbows are at 90-degree angles.

Exhale as you slowly and carefully push back off the wall to your starting position.

Repeat as many times as possible to increase your strength and endurance.

Decline Push-ups

Like with incline push-ups, you'll need an elevated surface, such as a bench or box, to do this activity. Recall that the workout will be more difficult when the surface is higher. If you are absolutely new to this activity, you should start with a low surface, such as a step, and gradually work your way up.

Begin by going down on all fours in front of the raised surface. Place your hands on the floor a little wider than shoulder width apart, fingers pointing forward.

Gently extend your legs one at a time to place your feet on the raised surface.
Strengthen your core and straighten your elbows so that your whole body straightens out and creates a long line from your head to your heels. Here is where your movement begins, often known as the beginning point.

Then, take a deep breath and bend your elbows to push yourself back into the floor in a calm and controlled manner until your arms form 90-degree angles.

Breathe out and push through your palm to return to the beginning position.

Push-ups on a Pike

Begin in a downward dog stance on the floor. Your hands should be shoulder-width apart and firmly planted on the floor. Your arms and legs should be straight, with your toes firmly pushed against the floor. Your body should create an upside-down V. Make sure your head is in line with your arms and your heels are slightly lifted off the ground. Next, carefully bend your elbows as you lower your upper body until your forehead almost meets the ground. Keep your legs straight.

Stop for 1 or 2 seconds, then straighten your arms and push yourself back up to the starting position.

This concludes one rep.

Formal hints

Your head should not contact or strike the floor, but it should be as near to the floor as feasible.

Push gently to prevent sliding, falling on your face, or damaging your shoulders.

Elevated pike push-ups

This action is identical to pike push-ups; the only difference is that you must lift your legs to make it more difficult.

Instructions: Go into the pike posture with your feet raised on a bench. Your hands should be shoulder-width apart and firmly planted on the floor. Your arms and legs should be straight, with your toes firmly placed on the bench. Bend your elbows gently as you lower your upper body until your forehead almost touches the ground.

Stop for 1 second, then push through your hands to return to the beginning pike position.

The Vertical Press

Vertical pressing is just lifting a weight in a straight line up and above. All of the exercises that utilize this movement pattern may be done with free weights like dumbbells and kettlebells or with your own body weight. My favorite exercise is the kettlebell single-arm military press.

Kettlebell one-arm military press

This can be done standing or sitting, but I'm showing you the standing form for now.

Begin by standing erect with a kettlebell in front of you. Stretch your knees and hips to grip the kettlebell with your right hand and bring it to your shoulder so that it is just above your shoulder. When you hoist the kettlebell, twist your wrist so that your palm faces inward. Keep your wrist straight and powerful; do not bend it. The kettlebell should also sit comfortably in the crook of your elbow, approximately chest height. This is the starting point.

Pinch your buttocks and brace your core to help balance your body. Look at the kettlebell and hoist it straight up without bouncing or bending your knees. Maintain a straight line with your wrist. Hold this posture for 1 or 2 seconds.

Continue the moves for a complete set, then transfer to the left hand.

Vertical press variations
Try them out from time to time since various approaches engage different portions of the same muscles, and it's also interesting to change up your routines.
Arnold pushes while standing with a kettlebell.

This Arnold Schwarzenegger version for the military press is always performed standing. This exercise targets the anterior delts more.

Instructions: Choose a kettlebell that you can lift easily without straining while still getting a good workout. Neither too light nor too hefty. Select one that allows you to comfortably execute roughly 10 reps.

Put the kettlebell directly in front of you on the floor.

Stretch your legs and hips to grip the kettlebell. Lift the kettlebell with one hand to your front delts, allowing it to rest precisely below your chin. Your arm should be at the peak of a biceps curl, palm facing inward. This is the starting point.

Maintain your wrist firm and straight, your elbow tucked into your sides, and your shoulders low and tight.

Open your arm and lift the kettlebell straight up while retracting your shoulders.

Lift the kettlebell overhead. When you raise the kettlebell overhead, twist your wrist so that your palm is facing away from you and stop for a second or two to generate strain on your delts. Gently descend the kettlebell in a controlled manner back to the beginning position and twist your wrist so that your palm faces you. If you are a novice or have physical restrictions that may make this movement pattern difficult, consider simpler alternatives, such as a modest shoulder press. If you want to make it more difficult, consider bodyweight options such as pike push-ups and bench pike push-ups.

Light shoulder press (1–5 pound weight)

Hold a dumbbell in one hand and stand tall with your legs shoulder-width apart.

The arm carrying the dumbbell should be bent at roughly a 60-degree angle, so that the dumbbell sits slightly above your shoulder and your palm faces your chest.

Maintain your core bracing and extend your elbow to raise the weight exactly over your head. Push it over your head until your arm is nearly entirely locked out.

Pause for a second or two, then gently drop the weight back to your shoulder in a controlled manner.

Rep for the recommended number of representatives.

The pull

Pulling exercises, like pushing exercises, may be done both horizontally and vertically. Rows are one of the horizontal pulling exercises. Pull exercises, like push exercises, help to build general upper-body strength.

Pull-ups are the most well-known pulling exercises, but I like to replace them with a single-arm kettle row since not everyone has a pull-up bar installed at home, and not every novice can execute many pull-ups in excellent form. Overall, all of these movements are excellent, and I prefer to use one or the other throughout my routine depending on the equipment available to me.

Kettlebell Row with Just One Arm

This exercise primarily works the back, posterior deltoid, lats, rhomboids, traps, and biceps.

Put a kettlebell in front of you.

Stand up straight with the kettlebell in front of you.

With your legs hip-width apart, take a big stride forward with your left leg to place your legs in a split stance.

To begin, slightly lean over. Your right leg and back should be straight, while your left knee should be bent to make a 90-degree angle.

For added support, place your left elbow on your left knee. Maintain a neutral spine.

Extend your right hand and grasp the kettlebell with a neutral grip.

This is the starting point.

Breathe out, then bend your elbow, retract your shoulder blade, and draw the kettlebell up towards your stomach. Keep your back straight.
Inhale as you drop the kettlebell back to the beginning position and repeat.
Complete all of the prescribed repetitions on the right side before moving to the left side.

Pull movements that alternate

Pull-up

Start by standing tall in front of a pullup bar.

Hold the bar with your hands facing away from you, shoulder width apart.
Hang from the bar with your arms fully extended. This is the starting point.
Lift yourself up. Squeeze your lats tight and bend your elbows, bringing them down toward the floor to lift yourself up.

Lift yourself up until your chin touches the bar. Stop for a second, then gently lower yourself down to the starting position. This completes one rep.

You could try negative pull-ups, TRX rows, or doorway rows if you are new to pulling exercises or if your body doesn't let you do pull-ups.

Complete Resistance Exercises (TRX)

I tried using TRX belts and resistance bands for exercises when I couldn't go to the gym due to quarantine, but I didn't enjoy them since I couldn't train all of my muscle groups properly with them. Yet, if you don't have a pull-up bar, these extras might be quite useful. You may perform standing rows with them:

Attach the TRX cable and resistance bands to something high so that the grips dangle at chest level.

Stand with your legs hip-width apart and hold the handles with both hands. Your hands should be facing each other.

Lean back and stretch your arms out to support your weight. The closer your feet are to the anchor, the more difficult the maneuver.

Raise yourself up to the handles so that they are directly under your sternum.
Maintain this posture for one second before inhaling and gently lowering yourself back to full extension.

This completes the first repetition.

Rows of doors

If you are traveling or do not have any resistance training equipment, you may practice this basic bodyweight row in a doorway.

Open the door you wish to use; stand in its path with your feet a few inches within the frame; grab onto its side frames with both hands at chest height; and lean back until your arms are completely extended. Bend your arms and drag yourself towards the door until your chest almost hits the doorway frames. This completes one repeat of the inverted row under the table.

Start by laying down beneath a sturdy table with your hands vertical to its edge, then fully extend your arms and hold the table's edge with an overhand grip. Your hands should be somewhat broader than shoulder width apart. Your fingers should be on the table's surface, and your heels should be on the ground. Make sure your body is hanging or slightly off the ground. Your heels should be the only portion of your body in contact with the floor.

Firm your core and squeeze your glutes to activate your lower back. Make sure your body is in a straight line from your torso to your feet.
Lift yourself up, leading with your chest, until it hits the table. During the exercise, keep your body straight, your core braced, and your glutes firm. Don't let your hips drop.

Maintain this posture for a second while ensuring your shoulder blades are retracted, then gently lower yourself back to the beginning position.

Keep in mind that, as simple as this exercise seems to be, carrying your weight with your fingers and doing a row action with your full body will require some skill. When I have a parallel bar handy, I like to complete this exercise with it.

The Base

Your core is made up of a group of complicated muscles that work together to support and bend the spine and run the whole length of your body on both the anterior and posterior sides.

When you do the main complex exercises properly, you work your core muscles heavily. This is why most individuals believe they do not need to conduct core workouts. But, if you look closely, you will see that most individuals who miss core workouts do not have remarkable midriffs.

The fact is that complex workouts, especially when performed with large weights, do not train all of your core muscles as much as people believe. Research has even confirmed this. That is why, in order to acquire the appearance you want, you must engage in a significant amount of exercise that targets your core. To strengthen your core, I suggest the following routines:

Leg Lifts

Lay on your back with your legs straight and your feet together. Your arms should be at your sides, palms facing down. Engage your core and straighten your legs as you raise them a few inches off the floor. Your toes should point away from your body, your pelvis should be somewhat tucked in, and your ribs should be down. Ensure to keep your chin tucked in during the action. This is the starting point.

While keeping that position, elevate your legs toward the sky by flexing your hips fully. Your legs and upper body should form a 90-degree angle.

Hold for one second at the apex of the movement.

Next, carefully lower your legs until they are barely over the ground.

Maintain this posture for a second before releasing.

Repeat for the prescribed number of repetitions.

Many core workouts

Leg lift while hanging

This exercise is not for everyone, and you will need a pull-up bar to complete it properly, but I feel it is the most effective exercise for training all portions of your abs.

Starting with an overhand hold on a pull-up bar, proceed with the instructions. Wrap your thumbs around the bar for more stability.

Engage your core by tightening your abs and hip flexors, and gently tilt your pelvis behind.

Raise your feet off the ground and extend your straight legs in front of you. At this part of the movement, exhale.

Continue lifting your legs as far as you can while maintaining proper form. Strive for lines parallel to the ground, or a little higher if feasible.

Maintain that posture for one second before inhaling and gently lowering your legs back to the starting position. This completes one repetition.

The Crack
Lay on your back with your knees bent, feet flat on the floor, and hips wide apart.
Put your hands behind your head, fingers clasped, and your elbows out to the sides.
In preparation for the exercise, brace your core and bring your navel towards your spine. Tilt your chin slightly to the side, leaving some space between it and your chest. This is the starting point.
Exhale as you curl up and forward, lifting your head, neck, and shoulder blades off the ground.
Hold at the top of the movement for a few seconds while breathing normally, and then slowly move back to the starting position.
Repeat while maintaining flawless form for each rep.

The Board

Begin by going down on all fours and putting your face down. Your elbows should be squarely under your shoulders, your toes should be anchored into the floor, and your forearms should be pointing forward. Maintain your head relaxed and your neck and spine neutralized by staring at a location on the floor approximately a foot beyond your hands.

Pull your navel inward and engage your core and abdominal muscles. Maintain a straight and firm torso. From your head to your toes, your complete body should be in a straight line. Maintain this posture for at least 15 seconds before releasing it to the floor.

As you get more comfortable with the maneuver, increase the holding duration.

Common grammatical errors

If you want to get the most out of your plank workout and keep your muscles from getting too tired and hurting you, don't do any of the following:
Your back is arched. An arched back stops you from using your core muscles, causing you to rely more on your arms. Keep your shoulders low and broad to prevent this.

Your hips are sagging. This occurs when your abs reach their limit of tiredness. This suggests you should put a stop to the plank. If your hips begin to droop at the beginning, attempt to spread your feet wider and focus on tightening your abdominals.

Tilting your head upward Avoid cocking your head. Maintain neutrality and alignment with the body. To avoid this, fix your gaze on a location on the floor.

And these are the six most crucial compound workouts that, when done correctly, will leave you never regretting a single resource put in here, whether it be time, effort, money, or anything else. You will obtain the physique of your dreams. Believe me!

Just follow all of the directions carefully and be certain of what you're doing. Further recommendations and aspects to consider in the next chapter will help you get the most out of these workouts.

The Fundamentals of Strength Training

Strength training is more than just lifting weights and pounding iron. Before you begin making any moves in the name of strength training, you must first learn a few methods. In this chapter, we'll go over all of the variables you should think about before starting your strength training program. Continue reading!

Frequency of Training

The frequency with which you exercise depends on a variety of variables, including your training objectives and degree of training. Frequent strength exercise stresses your muscles and causes some tissue microtrauma (a temporary weakness in muscle cells that stimulates tissue-building processes and strength development).

Following each workout, the worked-out tissues regenerate in response to the training stimulus. As a consequence, the muscles get stronger and bigger. This tissue-building process might take anywhere from a day to a week. While the frequency of your workout may vary, most experts suggest working most major muscle groups once every 3 to 5 days.

Individual exercises with increased intensity and volume might be done less often to allow for enough recovery time. You should also take several days off from exercise throughout the week to allow your muscles to properly heal. To ensure that I am completely healed, I always strive to rest for at least two days (48 hours) before resuming my training.

If you can lift weights three days a week, training for three nonconsecutive days per week with rest days in between (e.g., Monday-Wednesday-Friday) promotes consistency and generates outstanding results. Yet, research suggests that strength training two days per week (for example, Mondays and Thursdays) has almost the same muscular growth benefit as three days of strength training per week (Westcott, 2015). As a consequence, this is my suggested alternative for achieving the greatest outcomes with the least amount of effort:

Hence, whether you strength train twice a week or three times a week, your pace of muscle growth should be the same since training frequency isn't as crucial as taxing your muscles sufficiently during each session and getting adequate recovery in between bouts.

You may also acquire strength by exercising just one day per week, but research suggests that, although this frequency helps to retain muscle, it slows the pace of muscle growth by roughly 50%. (Westcott et al. 2009).

Some individuals segregate their muscle groups and go to the gym 3–6 times per week. That's just fine. If your aim for strength training is to maintain your strength and muscle, you may even perform 1 whole-body exercise every 2 weeks.

But I do not recommend missing your exercise for two weeks. Instead, I recommend completing 1-3 workouts a week to stay consistent, depending on how much your body can take, what you want to achieve with your physique, and how much time you have available for workouts.

Keep in mind that consistency is just as crucial as frequency. Skipping exercise sessions on your plan is inefficient, and strengthening your muscles without enough recuperation to compensate for missing days is counterproductive.

As a result, it is critical to develop a consistent every-other-day, every-other-two-days, or every-other-week strength training routine that is appropriate with your objectives, recuperation, and lifestyle and that involves 1 to 3 days of training each week.

Reps and Sets

A set of repetitions in a certain exercise is referred to as an exercise set. For example, if you take up a kettlebell and do 8 military presses before returning it, you've accomplished one set of 8 repetitions. You will have finished two sets of eight repetitions if you take a break and then resume this technique.

If you are just starting out with a strength training regimen, you should just do one set of each exercise. According to research, people who begin strength training may get the same muscle-building advantages by executing one set per exercise as they would by performing three sets.

This is because muscles react quicker to a resistance workout in untrained individuals since their strength level is always low when they begin exercising. There is still opportunity for improvement. Doing one set of each exercise at the start also helps you master the techniques and prevent injuries.

The good news is that this noticeable and immediate improvement inspires you to continue working out. But, as time passes (after 3 or 4 months), strength improvements plateau. And it is at this point that you should raise the number of sets and advance to 3 to 5 sets per exercise to get the required muscle improvement.

Reps, on the other hand, refer to the number of times you complete a certain strength-training activity in a single set. The ideal number of repetitions for each set is between 6 and 12. The top end of this spectrum emphasizes muscular endurance, while the lower end emphasizes strength and power.

Your muscles react differently depending on the stimulus you apply, such as modifying the number of repetitions completed each set, the weight or load being lifted, the number of sets, the duration under stress, or the pace at which you execute the activity.

The most essential thing to remember about repetitions per set is that you want to hit muscular failure within the 6–12 range or any other range of your choosing based on your primary aim for strength training, whether it is muscle endurance or strength and power.

If your main aim is to increase power and strength, you must only execute 1-6 reps, which means you cannot perform another rep after you reach 6 repetitions; you have hit muscular failure. If you can't perform one rep, the weight is too much for you. If you can do more than 6 repetitions, it suggests the weight is too light for your power and strength.

If muscular endurance is your main goal in strength training, you should be able to complete 12 or more repetitions. If you can't complete the 12th rep, the weight is too heavy for your muscles to handle.

To summarize, the number of sets completed in an exercise varies according to your training objectives. The National Strength and Conditioning Association (NSCA) recommends the following set range (Kamb, 2021):

If you want to improve muscle endurance, you should do 2-3 sets of 12 to 20+ repetitions.

If you want to increase muscle hypertrophy, you should do 3-6 sets of 6–12 repetitions.

If your aim is to increase muscle strength, you should execute 2–6 sets of fewer than 6 reps.

Keep in mind that these are the best ranges for building strength or muscle. It does not imply that if you execute four sets, you will only gain strength and not muscle, or that if you perform ten reps, you will only build muscle and not strength.

According to certain research, you may build the same muscles by completing numerous repetitions with smaller weights until failure. I favor the opposite approach: higher weights and fewer repetitions. For example, instead of 3x30, execute 3x10 repetitions. This saves time and allows you to concentrate on good body form and movement methods.

Based on the recommendations above, I recommend executing three sets of six to twelve repetitions to gain the advantages of both muscle and strength growth. Remember to choose a weight that is sufficiently difficult. If you can't complete 6 repetitions, the weight is too heavy, and if you can do more than 12 reps, it's time to obtain heavier weight or utilize alternative progression techniques (I will introduce them to you further in this chapter). Hence, if you can accomplish more than the maximum number of repetitions necessary to attain a given objective, it's time to increase the weight in order to develop your exercise.

My advice is to start with a weight that you can only lift six times. If you are not a total novice, it may take a year or more before you can perform more than 12 repetitions with this weight and need to replace it. Similarly, before raising the weight, you might attempt alternative strategies for progressing in your exercises.

Repetition Rate

The repetition speed relates to how quickly you raise and lower the weight in each repetition (weight, in this case, includes body weight too, and lift also refers to the upward movement of your weight regardless of the direction your body moves). In layman's terms, it is the amount of time necessary to complete each repetition.

The greater the duration under strain, the longer it takes to finish a rep or set. Slow down the activity if an exercise gets so simple that you can complete more repetitions than the maximum recommended. Spend more time concentrating while you push your muscles through their entire range of motion. This makes your muscles work harder, resulting in increased physical strength, endurance, and development.

Reduce your pace to maximize time under strain throughout your exercise. For example, completing the kettlebell goblet squat with a tempo of 1:1:1 involves taking one second to lower your body, one second to stop in the squat position, and one second to rise up and return to the starting position.

If the movement comes naturally to you, slow it down to a pace of 2:1:2, 3:1:3, and so on. Increase the weight you're using when you can easily finish the movements at a 5:1:5 speed.

While repeat pace varies depending on personal choice, it is critical to regulate all of your training repetitions. When we say "under control," we often mean repetition speed without the use of inertia or momentum (this is not the case for kettlebell swing). Controlled muscle tension both challenges your body and reduces your chance of damage.

The stop test is one of the finest techniques to evaluate your repetition speed. During a repeat, try halting at any position in the movement range. If you can stop, you're utilizing the appropriate repeat speed. Do this test throughout your exercises to see whether you're doing your repetitions at the correct pace.

Weight/Exercise Load

The first safety consideration for anybody engaged in strength training is always the selection of a proper workout resistance or load. The most crucial thing is to make sure your beginning weight is not excessive. The number of repetitions completed in an exercise set is mostly dictated by the amount of resistance used or the weight lifted.

If your primary goal is muscular strength, you should lift a weight that allows you to comfortably perform 1-6 reps. Continue to exercise with these weights until you can do more repetitions with the same loads, then raise or modify the resistance in accordance with the overload principle.

Rest intervals between sets and exercises

A rest period is the time spent between sets resting to enable your muscles to heal. The time between sets is generally between 30 seconds and 2 minutes (Rogers, 2020). Let your muscles recuperate for 1-2 minutes between sets while doing two or more sets of the same activity. This time is adequate to recuperate your muscles and replenish the majority of the energy utilized in completing the actions.

You should also take a short break between workouts to lessen the overall impact of exhaustion on your physical efforts. 1-2 minutes of rest between workouts is generally sufficient.

For various training purposes, the rest duration between exercise sets often falls within the following ranges:

The rest period between sets should be 2 to 5 minutes if you want to improve muscular strength.

The rest period between sets during an activity should be 30 to 60 seconds if you want to build muscular endurance.

If muscular growth is your aim, then the rest period between workout sets should be 30 to 90 seconds.

After completing your workout, you may rest until your breathing returns to normal before going on to the next. That's exactly what I do. I don't always pace myself to make sure I'm resting for precisely 1-2 minutes between workouts.

Pattern of Breathing

Never hold your breath when strength training, regardless of the kind or intensity of the activity. Holding your breath might result in increased internal pressure, which can limit blood flow. This may cause symptoms such as lightheadedness and high blood pressure reactions, interfering with your exercise. Breathe consistently during your training sessions to avoid these negative consequences.

Exhale at the sticking point, which is the hardest part of each repetition (hard lifting, pushing, or pulling), and inhale during the easier lowering or return phase. a more optimal internal pressure response. Since continuous breathing is a vital component of safe strength training activities, you should practice appropriate breathing on every repetition during the whole workout.

Body Shape

Proper body posture during exercise is more essential than the weights lifted or the sets and reps performed. Perfecting your form throughout the exercises will help you enhance your game and body. These are some of the advantages of exercising with excellent form: It aids in the prevention of injuries. Proper form throughout exercises helps you prevent weight- and flexibility-related issues. Lifting weights (whether your own body weight, free weight, or any other) exerts extra strain on your muscles. And since all of your bodily components are interconnected, if one goes out of balance, the rest suffer. For example, if you squat incorrectly, you run the risk of damaging your back.

It aids in the reduction of energy lost during exercise. Bad form during a workout leads you to exert more effort and energy while doing the exercises. When you exercise properly, you may use significantly less energy to complete the same workout. Your exercise becomes easier and more pleasant! There will be no straining.

It improves the efficacy and efficiency of workouts. Proper form during an activity provides a beneficial workout experience. It allows you to move your joints and muscles through their entire range of motion, resulting in total muscular extension and contraction and hence greater outcomes.

Despite the fact that the words 'posture' or 'form' may seem common and basic, most individuals do not do their workouts in perfect bodily form. Nonetheless, you should be aware that appropriate form is critical to reaching your fitness objectives. It reduces muscular tension and provides a pain-free environment for activity. It also allows you to work the specific muscles appropriately.

Motion Possibility

A range of motion refers to how far your joints can move on each exercise. In other words, it refers to your joints' capacity to perform the whole range of motions throughout an activity. The majority of doctors advocate exercising over the whole range of joint mobility. I also endorse it. According to research, training your body over its whole range of motion is essential for establishing full-range physical strength.

Exercising from complete muscle stretch to full muscular contraction is referred to as "full range of motion." When the target muscle group is completely stretched, the opposing muscle group is fully contracted, and vice versa.

Your biceps and triceps are an excellent example; if you move your elbow joint through its complete range of motion, your biceps stretch fully while your triceps contract fully. Of course, you should not push your joints beyond their natural limitations or experience discomfort during any part of the action. Avoid any activity that produces joint pain or discomfort, and only train in a range of motion that is pain-free.

Exercise with a wide range of motion provides the following advantages:

Improves joint flexibility. Exercising over the whole range of motion enhances joint flexibility. When it comes to exercising your body, flexibility is essential since it assists with posture and weight lifting during strength training. As a result, if you want your exercise to be more effective and efficient, you must go across the whole range of motion.

Allows you to do more workouts with less effort. Exercising in a broad range of joint mobility helps you do more difficult workouts while using less energy. According to research, those who exercise their muscles over their whole range of motion enhance their muscular strength, allowing them to carry higher weights without effort.

Improves the development of full-range muscular strength. The weights you lift and how you lift them are crucial to muscle gain. Lifting your weight through the whole range of joint motion improves strength in all muscles, according to research (Westcott, 2015). Lowering the range of motion in a workout reduces muscular tension, which inhibits muscle development. Lifting heavier weights, on the other hand, stimulates your muscle fiber, which increases the number of muscle cells in your body, boosting growth. To improve muscular strength and power, you must exercise over the whole range of motion.

Progression of Exercise

Most of us aspire for workout growth. Nonetheless, some people will always do what is most comfortable for them, such as complete the same reps or sets with the same weight. This is in opposition to the increasing overload concept, which is the primary training principle.

According to the progressive overload concept, in order to continue developing strength and muscle mass or to accomplish any other exercise-related gains, you must gradually raise your muscles' working load in order to consistently push your body and muscles with new training stimuli.

Keep in mind that not all workouts improve at the same pace. Again, don't pack on the pounds too quickly, and don't push development by losing form. Instead, you will do more harm to your body.

Despite the fact that this is the most typical technique for transitioning from one session to the next, many individuals do it incorrectly. It's not about how much weight you can lift. What is most important is that you do it correctly.

To prevent injuries and achieve excellent outcomes, lift a lesser weight in full range of motion repetitions rather than half-sloppy reps with greater loads. I'm not saying half reps and greater weights are bad. No. That is, it is correct and safer to perfect your form using the full-range version first.

To increase your weight, utilize a larger load while maintaining the same repetitions, sets, rest time, and pace. For example, if you are presently lifting 50 pounds on a certain exercise, you may increase your weight to 52.5 pounds the following time you do the same exercise. According to research, increasing your weight load by as little as 2.5 pounds at each level of training progression is both safe and beneficial. But, when using a single dumbbell or kettlebell, this is not as straightforward, thus I favor alternative progression approaches.

Additional Ways of Advancement

I've previously discussed how you may speed up your improvement by raising your weights or time under stress. Several progression strategies may be used to ensure that you are continually progressing toward your fitness goals:

Increase the number of sets. To advance your sets, add one set while keeping the weight and rest time the same. For example, if you lift 50 pounds for three sets of ten repetitions on one exercise, you may perform four sets of ten reps the following time.

Increase your reps. To increase your reps, add one rep to each set while keeping the weight and rest time the same. For example, if you're lifting 50 pounds for three sets of five repetitions on one exercise, you may attempt three sets of six reps with the same weight the following time you complete the same program.

Reducing your rest time. While reducing your rest between sets, strive to keep the weight and reps/sets the same. This makes the activity more difficult. For example, if you normally rest for 2 minutes between sets while executing a certain exercise, reduce the rest period to 1 minute and 30 seconds while lifting the same weight for the same number of repetitions and reps.

What counts most during strength training is how we perform our workouts. To obtain the physical and emotional advantages of your exercise, you must consider all of the aspects listed above. You should be primarily concerned with appropriately doing the exercises presented in order to develop the muscle memory and technique necessary for long-term benefits. To do this, just follow the advice and recommendations offered in this book.

With a practical grasp and respect for these training concepts, I feel you're now ready to follow the basic exercise regimen I've devised for you in the next chapter. Remember that in order to continue progressing in your exercises, you must maintain the appropriate training intensity, which is influenced by the concepts discussed above.

Important Takeaways

While doing your exercise, keep good form and posture in mind. While lifting weights, make sure your joints move through their complete range of motion, and never hold your breath while exercising. Exhale at the most difficult portion of each repetition (tough lifting, pushing, or pulling) and inhale during the gentler lowering or return phase.

Give your muscles 1–2 minutes of rest between sets and activities so they can recover.

To get the most out of your training, do 3 sets of 6–12 repetitions of each exercise.

Strive for two workouts each week to get the greatest benefits with the least amount of effort.

The Extreme Workout Plan

I hope this book has been beneficial thus far and that you've gained some ideas, insights, or views to help you get started on your strength training adventure. Exercises cannot become a workout until they are planned and organized into a program, and a workout program cannot assist you in meeting your training objectives unless it is simple to follow, imaginative, and successful.

And I've done exactly that in this chapter. Nevertheless, before we get started on the training regimen, let's talk about muscle preparation before a workout and cooling down afterward. We'll also do our workouts in supersets, about which I'm sure you'd want to know what they are and why we're utilizing them in our program.

Warm-up and cool-down periods

It might be tempting to forgo a warm-up at times, particularly if you are pressed for time or just eager to begin your exercise. Warming up before participating in rigorous physical exercise, on the other hand, offers very genuine physiological and psychological advantages.

Strength training is one of the toughest exercises that puts a significant strain on your musculoskeletal system. As a result, it is critical to warm up before beginning strength training. Jogging in place, brisk walking, and jumping rope are excellent techniques to rapidly warm up for your activity. These warm-up exercises should only take 2–5 minutes to complete.

The Advantages of Warming Up

Reduces the possibility of harm. Sprains, strains, and other types of injuries are the last thing you should experience after working out consistently. Warming up your muscles improves their suppleness, lowering your risk of injury or overheating during activity. Mentally prepares you for what is to come. As your training becomes more challenging, it is quite easy to lose motivation and give up. You are less likely to do so if you warm up before the activity. This is due to the fact that when you warm up, your brain concentrates on your body and the physical activity; this attention continues over into your training session, reminding you of your workout objectives.

Improves adaptability. Warm-ups relax your muscles, making it simpler to move and do your program correctly. Increases blood flow and oxygen levels. A 5-minute warm-up with an easygoing exercise such as jogging in place dilates blood vessels, increasing blood flow to your skeletal muscles. This helps supply your muscles with the needed quantity of oxygen during activity, therefore eliminating what we sometimes term "oxygen debt". It is just as vital to cool down after a workout as it is to warm up. The main goal of cooling down after exercise is to slowly get your heart rate and blood pressure back to normal. This is just a warm-up in reverse.

During the workout, your heart has been beating harder and faster than usual. It is important to slowly get back to normal instead of stopping all of a sudden.

The cool-down is especially important for older people because it keeps blood and other body fluids from building up in the lower legs, which could cause blood pressure changes and heart problems. A 5- to 10-minute cool-down activity, like brisk walking followed by stretching, helps the blood flow and heart rate get back to normal.

The Importance of Cooling Off

It promotes muscular repair. Lactate builds up in the blood after strenuous activity, making it acidic. This causes lactic acid to accumulate in your musculoskeletal system. It takes time for this lactic acid to leave your body. As a result, cooling-down workouts assist in the process of lactic acid release and removal, resulting in faster muscle recovery.

Reduces DOMS (delayed onset muscle soreness). While muscle soreness after an exercise is natural, a substantial quantity of DOMS may cause pain and hinder you from exercising in the future. According to research, cooling down after an exercise helps eliminate excessive muscular discomfort, making you feel more at ease and prepared for the next session.

Stretching
It's a good idea to stretch. Even if you don't exercise often, stretching should be part of your daily regimen. It keeps your muscles supple and allows them to move through their full range of motion. The American College of Sports Medicine suggests stretching each of your main muscle groups for 60 seconds at least twice a week (Collins, 2012).

Should you stretch before you exercise?

Static stretching should not be done before an activity. There is no evidence that static stretching before exercise may help avoid injury, reduce post-exercise muscular soreness, or increase performance. In fact, studies suggest that exercising static stretching alone before working out may reduce muscular strength and power, as well as impair performance (Simic, 2013). Instead, warm up by doing active stretches.

Should you stretch after you exercise?

This is an excellent time to stretch. Static stretching after exercise allows you to cool down, recoup, and prepare for the next workout. Stretching during this time will assist in the delivery of nutrients and oxygen to the damaged muscles, aiding in recuperation and regeneration. It also aids in the relaxation of your neurological system and the slowing of your pulse rate.

Stretching carefully

If you must stretch before your exercise, make sure your muscles are not fully cold. Warm-up exercises should be performed before stretching to help produce heat in your muscles. Shaking portions of your body, such as your arms, hands, and legs, may help you do this. Hold the static stretch for at least 30 seconds if it is done after a workout. Let your body adjust to the extension. This is much better for your tissues. Try pushing harder when you're on the verge. You should not feel any discomfort throughout the stretch. If you do, you're doing it incorrectly and should quit. Take your time and do it well.

Supersets

This basically means doing two separate workouts back-to-back with extremely little break in between.

The Advantages of Supersets

They help you save time. When you're short on time, supersets are ideal. Performing two separate exercises without or with little rest periods between them shortens and increases the efficiency of your workout. I can do my whole-body exercise in 30 minutes by using supersets.

Intensity has been increased. Supersets allow you to do more work in less time, which allows you to get more out of your training regimen.

Increases muscular endurance. Supersets strengthen your muscles to operate for extended periods of time. They aid in the development of strength and endurance, as well as the burning of more calories. Numerous studies have shown that supersets increase calorie expenditure during and after a workout.

Improve active rest. When you do supersets, you train one muscle while resting the opposite one. This increases muscular building while decreasing body fat.

The Scheme

When it comes to muscle development training, one of the most essential things to practice is the best compound exercises—the actual core muscle building motions given in Chapter 4. You must also improve in these areas.

Especially if you are over 40 or 50, you need to do these workouts every day as part of a set program if you want to get better. After we've learned how to do the compound movements, we need to know how often we should practice. Frequency just means how often we work a muscle part, and there are many ways to work out to build muscle. Each one has its own set of advantages.

The majority of the time, you'll find in these bodybuilding publications that they propose you break up your training regimen, such as only doing chest on Monday, back on Tuesday, shoulders on Wednesday, legs on Thursday, and arms on Friday. There are really sophisticated split routines, and it turns out that with this training technique, you do a ton of sets for chest on Monday and then don't touch chest for another five to seven days. It is not the best approach for most of us to train. What I recommend is a higher-frequency workout with fewer sets per session. That is, instead of completing a lot of sets on Monday for chest, split those sets over 2 to 3 sessions by training chest 2 to 3 days each week with enough rest in between.

When you exercise a muscle, you receive a protein synthesis muscle-building stimulus a few days later after the training session that only lasts a couple days, and then you have to train again to obtain that stimulus. We don't get significantly more protein synthesis if we pound our chest for 20 sets than if we simply completed a few strong sets. When we perform 20 sets per muscle group, we just build additional roadblocks to healing and retain that pain. Then we won't be able to workout for another five to seven days.

When we go into our 40s and 50s, it's even more important to spread out that volume even more with 2 to 3 full-body sessions each week that include all of the finest compound exercises. It is because we do the ideal amount of sets and have adequate time to recuperate. As you hit the body more often, the muscle-building stimulation remains consistent. Hence, for effective training, the correct kind of workouts and volume are critical.

I've incorporated workouts that are incredibly effective on their own in the regimen below. This program increases efficacy while reducing effort, resulting in incredible outcomes.

Helpful Hints

Perform push-ups and goblet squats without rest (superset #1). After doing these two exercises once, rest for 1-2 minutes before repeating superset #1. After completing superset #1 three times, pause for 1-2 minutes before proceeding to supersets #2, #3, and #4. I recommend that you do 6–12 repetitions of each exercise.

I started with push-ups and squats because they are simple, work a lot of muscles, and are a great way to warm up.I saved swing for last since it's the riskiest for novices, and I want you to be thoroughly warmed up after the other three supersets. While supersets may help you complete your workout quicker, you can also perform standard sets: do one exercise for three sets with a 1-2 minute break between sets, and then go on to the next exercise. Chapter 4 discusses these and all other essential exercises. There you will also discover all of the other workouts you can substitute for any of my suggested routines.

But, it is crucial to understand that there are other methods to build your training program, and what I have here is not always consistent. You may alter it and change it to meet your training objectives. But if you want to get fantastic results with no effort, this might be a terrific and sustainable training strategy for you, as it is for me.

If you have a barbell, a pull-up bar, or parallel bars close by, you might want to include exercises that use them in your routine. When I can, I like to use this equipment to do exercises like incline bench press instead of push-ups or pull-ups instead of rows. So don't be surprised if you can't get your hands on this stuff. The most essential thing is to execute the complex workouts listed above with whatever equipment is available, or even without one. Both the dumbbell and the kettlebell are excellent tools for increasing personal fitness. If you have a pair of dumbbells, you can do the following complex movements:

Dumbbell Workout Routine

1. Dumbbell Swing as a Hinge (or Dumbbell Deadlift)
2. Pull: Dumbbell Row with One Arm (or Two-Arm Dumbbell Row)
3. Dumbbell Bench Press Push-up (or Incline Dumbbell Bench Press)
4. Squats using dumbbells (or dumbbell lunges)
5. Seated Dumbbell Press Vertical Press (or Standing Dumbbell Press)

Leg Lift is a core exercise (or Crunch, Plank).

If you have some strength training experience or are returning to resistance training after a break, an above-intermediate exercise plan with free weights will most likely be the best match for you. Can novices use kettlebells and dumbbells to train?

Yeah, without a doubt. Beginners may exercise with free weights without difficulty; however, while utilizing them for the first few sessions, form should take priority over attention. If you're new to exercising, recuperating from an injury, prefer low-intensity strength training, or have physical restrictions that may hinder movement patterns, I suggest beginning with beginner workout programs that use smaller weights, resistance bands, or solely bodyweight exercises.

Anyone who wants to tone their muscles, keep their strength up, and improve their overall health can do bodyweight exercises or exercises with resistance bands at home or on the go. These exercises are a wonderful resource not only for seniors wishing to enhance their strength and body composition without purchasing a gym but also for bodybuilders searching for a difficult training session when the gym is out of reach.

Not everyone who wants to grow stronger and fitter can or wants to go to the gym. Maybe they don't have time. Maybe the cost of a gym membership is out of their budget, or they are uncomfortable in a gym setting and would rather work up a sweat in the privacy of their own home. If this is the case for you, a bodyweight training regimen is an excellent choice.

Bodyweight Exercise Routine

1. Hip Lift Hinge (or Standing Back Extensions)
2. Bodyweight rowing (or doorway rows)
Knee push-ups are a type of push-up (also known as Wall, Incline, and Decline Push-ups).
4. Squat: Squats with Bodyweight (or Chair, Box Squats, Bodyweight Lunge)
5. Pike push-up vertical press (or Incline Pike Push-up)
6. Leg Lift While Laying (or Crunch, Plank)

Routine Exercise with Resistance Bands

1. Hinge: Resistance Band Deadlift
2. Pull: Rows with resistance bands
3. Push-ups: Push-ups using a resistance band
4. Squats using resistance bands
5. Vertical Press with Resistance Band: Vertical Press with Resistance Band
6. Leg Lift While Laying (or Crunch, Plank)

When you get stronger as you progress and feel like you need something more challenging to challenge your muscle strength, or if you've had a lot of experience with bodyweight training or weightlifting and are looking for more challenging weights and workouts, advanced exercises with a barbell are likely to suit you best.

While barbell exercises are not for everyone, many people think that they are the foundation of the finest strength training regimens since bigger weights help you grow muscle and strength quicker than anything else. Although this is sufficient to advance on most bodyweight or equipment-based exercises, it may not be sufficient to accomplish progressive overload on movements like the squat, deadlift, bench press, and dumbbell row after many years of adequate training. Thus, if you're a seasoned lifter who wants or can go to the gym, these are the finest barbell workouts to increase strength and muscle mass:

Routine for Barbell Workouts
1. Barbell Deadlift Hinge
2. Pull: bent-over row with barbell (or pull-up)
3. Push-up: Bench Press with a Barbell (or Incline Barbell Bench Press)
4. Squat: Back squat with a barbell (or barbell front squat).
5. Vertical Press: Overhead Barbell Press (or Military Press)

Core: Leg Lift in the Air (or Incline Crunch, Plank)

Important Takeaways

Always warm up before beginning your exercise. Utilizing supersets is a terrific method to save time.
Concentrate on compound motions rather than specific exercises or equipment; altering one or more exercises or pieces of equipment from time to time can make your workouts more effective and enjoyable.

Important Nutrients

Activity and nutrition are inextricably linked. You can never debate one while ignoring the other. If you want to have a healthy, strong, and attractive figure, you must not only exercise but also eat properly.

Eating healthy does not have to mean eating just salads and boring things. Your diet should not feel more like a form of self-denial than self-improvement.

What I'm trying to express is that you can have a solid diet plan based on the things you like. You don't have to give up your favorite meals in order to follow the "clean eating" trend.

The diet you choose will be determined by your fitness goals. If you want to lose weight, you should eat fewer calories; if you want to gain weight and muscle mass, you should consume more calories. It's simply basic biology; but, what I've learned through the years is that you don't have to starve yourself to lose weight, and you don't have to eat yourself every time you gain weight or muscle mass. Someone with a clear head would see that both of these viewpoints are potentially lethal.

To begin, you should be aware that various individuals have varied body types and metabolic processes. A diet plan that works for someone else may not work for you. As a result, while attempting to develop an eating regimen, arrange it differently than you are used to.

For example, if you want to reduce weight and you usually eat four meals a day, cut one of them down to three.

So, when we boil it all down, it comes down to moderation, controlled, and scheduled eating. Regardless of your training objectives, you should limit your intake of processed and sugary "foods" to a minimum.

So, there's this argument going on about what's most essential in fitness. Exercise or nutrition? Some feel that exercise is the most significant component, while others argue that it is secondary to food and other variables. Others still claim that one is 40% and the other is 60%. If you didn't already know, diet is really essential.

Do I sound insane? You're probably wondering what percentage exercise has. Exercise is also 100 percent.

Note that there are additional elements, but these two are the most important. Does that sound strange? I understand your confusion regarding the entire percentage. Indeed, it can go all the way up to 1,000 percent. The argument is that the components of a magnificent physique are more like pillars than jigsaw pieces. If one is too weak, the whole building falls. You must provide your body with sufficient nourishment in order for it to adapt to your workout. Therefore, in order to build more muscle and strength, you must workout properly.

If you continue to consume a lot of nutrient-empty calories without the proper macronutrient balance, your strength training efforts will be futile.

Macronutrients and micronutrients

Micronutrients are vitamins and minerals. Our bodies need certain vitamins and minerals to function properly. They aid in the control of metabolism, heart rate, and bone density. Proteins, carbs, and lipids are examples of macronutrients. To operate properly, our bodies need a balance of micro- and macronutrients.

Proteins

Proteins are well-known for their ability to build muscle and increase strength. As we get older, our testosterone levels drop, as does our muscular mass. As a consequence, fat cells may take the place of muscle cells, resulting in an unwanted weight gain or body shape change and weak muscles. You will need to eat more protein if you want to gain muscle mass.

Moreover, as we age, our metabolism slows, and even healthy seniors need more protein than they did when they were younger to help keep muscle mass. As a result, it is advised that you eat 1.2–1.7 grams of protein per kilogram of your target body weight or 0.5–0.8 grams per pound of your target body weight every day.

Protein-rich foods include fish, eggs, lean meat, beans, and soybean products such as tofu.

Carbohydrates Choose complex carbohydrates over simple carbohydrates. To stay healthy, avoid simple carbs like added sugars and processed grains, which are high in empty calories. Complex carbohydrates may be found in meals such as oatmeal, whole grains, legumes (beans and lentils), sesame seeds, and so on.

Fat

Dietary fat is vital because it provides energy and aids in food absorption as well as nervous system function. Saturated and unsaturated fats are the two kinds of fats. The difference between the two is that unsaturated fats are liquid at room temperature and are regarded as the healthiest, while saturated fats are solid.

Certain unsaturated fatty acids are necessary nutrients, which means our bodies cannot produce them and we must get them from diet. Nevertheless, certain meals, such as meat and poultry proteins, may include unsaturated fats, so be cautious when picking them and cut visible fats.

Choose unsaturated fats over saturated fats to reduce your risk of stroke and cardiovascular disease. Nuts like cashew and almond, as well as avocado, are high in healthy fats. These fats are unsaturated. Foods high in saturated fats, such as fatty meats and shortening, should be avoided.

Nutrition Before and After Exercise

It is essential that you pay close attention to your pre- and post-workout diet. A good diet before and after exercise helps you balance your glucose levels, recover properly and quickly, and improve your performance. As a result, it is essential to select a diet that is appropriate for your body and may effectively complement your training schedule.

Nutrition for Pre-Workout

Before you begin exercising, you must feed your body with the appropriate nutrients in the appropriate amounts based on your training objective. This not only guarantees that your body has the energy to keep lifting weights during the activity, but it also improves your performance.

As a result, before your training, ingest meals that will provide you with enough energy to complete your final activity. Proteins and carbohydrates should be included in the meal.

Each of these macronutrients has a distinct purpose. Their intake ratio, however, fluctuates according to your training aim and the sort of activity. For example, if your objective is to lose weight, you will need to eat fewer carbohydrates and more proteins before your activity. If you want to build muscle, your pre-workout meal should include more proteins and carbohydrates in larger portions.

Let's take a look at the responsibilities that each of these macronutrients performs before exercising:

Carbs
Carbohydrates provide fuel for your muscles throughout your activity. The more and harder you workout, the more carbohydrates you will need to stay going. Carbohydrates aid in weight management and offer the energy required to do the activities. Recall that your muscles need glucose from carbohydrates to power

your body during exercise. That is why "good" carbohydrates are necessary in your pre-workout diet.

A "healthy" carb to ingest before your exercise is bananas, oats, or whole grains. It is suggested that you ingest 0.25–0.5 grams of carbohydrates per pound of body weight 3–4 hours before your exercise. But, keep in mind that this number lowers as you get closer to your exercise. For example, if you have to eat one hour before your exercise, you will only require 0.25 grams of carbohydrates per pound of body weight.

Proteins
Who doesn't know that proteins help develop muscle? Proteins are widely recognized for their ability to construct and repair our bodies. Numerous studies have shown that eating protein before working out boosts muscle protein synthesis. It also promotes anabolic response, increases muscular strength and mass, and boosts performance and muscle recovery.

Yogurt or protein smoothies are excellent pre-workout beverages. It is suggested that you ingest 20 grams of protein before working out. Do you want to know how soon you should eat before working out? Preferably, you should feed your body the nutrients listed above 1–3 hours before your activity. But, if you want to optimize your results, you should have a comprehensive breakfast with proteins, fats, and some carbohydrates 2-3 hours before your exercise.

If you can't have a complete meal within this time frame for any reason, you can still eat something good. A snack may also be beneficial. But if you must eat too soon before exercising, the food should be easy to digest and modest in size.

The following are some of the best things to eat before working out:

Oatmeal made with low-fat milk

Banana and mixed berries Whole grain bread, eggs, and brown rice sandwich with lean protein and veggies

Greek yogurt with fruits Whole-grain cereal, a protein smoothie, and chicken breast

Nutrition After Exercise

Don't forget about your post-workout diet while you focus on your pre-workout nutrition. It is just as crucial to eat the correct foods after working out as it is before. To understand why it is necessary to consume the correct foods in the proper ratios and proportions, you must first understand how physical exercise affects your body.

I'll explain what occurs in a nutshell: During exercise, your muscles deplete glycogen reserves in order to feed your body. This causes your muscles' glycogen reserves to be partially depleteds deplete glycogen reserves in order to feed your body. This causes your muscles' glycogen reserves to be partially depleted. Remember that your body needs glucose to function normally. As a result, after exercise, your body must rebuild, repair, and regenerate muscle proteins, as well as restore depleted glycogen reserves.

As a result, after working out, you should take meals that will aid in this process. As a result, your post-workout food should include lots of protein as well as some carbohydrates. They suggest eating your post-workout meals within 45 minutes after finishing your workout. Therefore, the earlier you eat, the better.

After an exercise, a balanced meal with protein and carbohydrates will restore your glycogen levels and aid in muscle development and repair. Consuming 20–40 grams of protein after exercise has also been shown in studies to improve muscle recovery time. Lean meat is the finest source of protein. Eggs are another excellent choice. It is also advised that you ingest 0.5–0.7 grams of carbohydrates per pound of body weight after your exercise. Oatmeal, potatoes, brown rice, fruits (banana, pineapple, and berries), and chocolate are some of the finest carbohydrates to ingest. If your main objective is to reduce weight, you may forego carbohydrates after your exercise and have roughly 40 grams of protein in total.

Following your workout, you may consume the following foods: Grilled chicken with roasted vegetables Low-fat yogurt with berries oatmeal, wheat flakes, cereal with fruits and nuts salmon with sweet potato Egg omelet with whole-grain toast and a burrito with green beans Chicken salad with mixed greens tofu with mushrooms brown rice with tenderloin steak

If you eat enough amounts of all macronutrients at breakfast, lunch, and dinner, it is also advisable to schedule your exercises between these meals or before your next meal. If the time between your exercise and meals is too lengthy, try consuming protein- and carbohydrate-rich snacks or supplements.

Supplements
When it comes to fitness, just try your best to get all of your nutrients from meals. Supplements are not as significant as many people believe. In truth, supplements are not required to reach your fitness objectives. But the appropriate ones might help you get results faster. Scientific evidence shows that some supplements may help you grow muscle and reduce fat quicker, increase your performance and muscle recovery, and improve your overall health. That is why you should think about including a few vitamins in your training routine.

Creatine, beta-alanine, and citrulline, for example, have been shown to help increase muscular development and strength quicker. Synephrine and yohimbine have also been demonstrated in studies to help you burn more fat. Vitamin D and fish oil, on the other hand, increase your health and well-being.

Another book would be required if I were to break down everything you see on the shelves of your local supplement shop. As a result, I'm only going to concentrate on a few supplements that have been shown to be the most effective in helping you achieve your health and fitness goals: fish oil, vitamin D, protein powder, a fat burner, and a muscle builder.

You may have a good and substantial impact on your health by using these five kinds of supplements. With these supplements, you may increase muscle growth and strength, shed weight, strengthen your immunity, improve your general health, and do much more. Let's take a closer look at them all.

1. Fatty fish oil

Fish oil is exactly what it sounds like: fish oil. Popular sources include salmon and sardines. Fish oil is high in omega-3 fatty acids, which are critical for muscle growth. These vital fatty acids are also required by our systems to avoid sickness.

According to research, the typical diet supplies barely one-tenth of these fatty acids. That is why supplements may be beneficial. Higher amounts of omega-3 fatty acids have been found to: decrease depression, anxiety, and stress; reduce muscular and joint discomfort; prevent you from accumulating extra fat; boost excess fat reduction; and improve cognitive ability.

2. D vitamin

Vitamin D is required for good bone health. It aids calcium absorption and may help prevent osteoporosis. It is also important in physiological processes such as metabolism, immune system function, and cell growth and development. This suggests that a lack of vitamin D might cause major health concerns.

Vitamin D is obtained from food, sunlight, or supplementation. Vitamin D is naturally found in a few foods, including cow liver, cheese, and egg yolk, albeit in very minute amounts. The majority of individuals acquire their vitamins from sunshine, but, as we age, our bodies' capacity to convert the sun's rays to vitamin D diminishes. As a result, supplementation becomes the most convenient and dependable method of increasing vitamin D levels in your body.

Regarding other vitamin supplements, most individuals do not need them and may get all of the vitamins and minerals they require by eating a healthy, balanced diet.

3. Body Fat Burner

I don't think I need to say anything further at this point. But I'll say it anyway: no medication or powder on the planet can make you healthier, stronger, or more attractive. That, believe it or not, is the harsh reality. Take it free of charge from me.

There is no "fat-burning" chemical that is safe and strong enough on its own to help people lose a lot of fat.Anybody offering to sell you such things is attempting to defraud you. Don't squander hundreds of dollars a month on useless pills marketed to steroid-fueled bodybuilders.
It's also not surprising that the majority of bodybuilding and weight-loss products on the market are duds. However, there are a few supplements that may help you accomplish your weight reduction target faster if you know how to drive it properly with the correct food and exercise. Caffeine is one of the few substances that has been confirmed by study to be useful in this field.

4. Muscle developers

Some individuals get dissatisfied after spending a lot of money on muscle-building pills that do not provide decent results. At this point, you should be aware that the majority of popular pills on the market that promise to help with muscle growth are completely ineffective. Thankfully, research has shown that a number of them are successful. Creatine is one of the few supplements that may help you grow muscle faster.

5. Protein Powder

If you are having difficulty getting enough protein in your diet for one reason or another, you may want to consider investing in an excellent protein powder (for example, you could be allergic to most of them). There are several protein powders available on the market, including vegan-friendly options. They exist to guarantee that you are obtaining enough proteins to adequately grow your muscles. Just add a scoop to your favorite beverage and you're ready to go! 20 grams of whey protein might also be beneficial when ingested before or after exercise.

Hydration

Water is very important to the human body. Water makes up around 70% of your body weight. Exercise accelerates the pace at which our bodies lose water. We lose a lot of water and electrolytes via sweat during and after exercise.

So, if you want to reach your fitness goals, you need to include a healthy way to stay hydrated in your training plan. Keeping hydrated is not only necessary during exercise; it is also necessary in our daily lives. "Water is life," they say. Insufficient fluid consumption causes dehydration, which may disrupt your body's normal functioning. Dehydration is the loss of bodily fluids and electrolytes. Without these critical components, your body cannot operate correctly.

Dehydration during exercise might reduce performance since it makes you feel tired and lethargic during your workout. It might also cause muscular cramps and headaches. Moreover, working out while dehydrated increases the danger of losing muscle endurance and strength.

The significance of bodily hydration

It improves your exercise performance. Dehydration may cause weariness, muscular cramps, decreased motivation, and changes in body temperature. All of this makes physical and mental activity seem more challenging. Consuming enough water and other vital fluids helps avoid dehydration, making exercise more enjoyable. Water helps digestion by breaking down food faster and making it easier for the body to absorb nutrients before and after exercise. Water and other fluids are great ways to get back the minerals and electrolytes that we lose when we sweat. Joints can move through their full range of motion when they are lubricated, which happens when you drink enough water. Water may also be used as a shock absorber.

Water also aids with weight reduction. Numerous studies have shown that drinking a glass of water before a meal reduces hunger and increases metabolism, assisting in weight reduction. Adequate hydration aids in the health of your skin. I'll remind you that you should drink 8 glasses of water every day, which comes to 2 liters.

Important Takeaways

Healthy dieting does not have to mean denying yourself what you want and eating bland meals. You can acquire and remain in shape while eating things you like.

Different people have different dietary needs based on their body type, age, and exercise goals.

Work with what you already have when creating a diet plan. Pre-exercise meals should be had 2-3 hours before your workout.

Eat your post-exercise meals within 45 minutes after finishing your workout. The sooner you start, the better.

If you eat a healthy diet, you won't require supplements. Strive to acquire as much of your nutrients from whole foods as possible; no pill or powder can make you healthier, stronger, or more attractive.

(For additional information on nutrition, see my books "Healthy Eating for Men" or "The Macros Diet Cookbook.")

The importance of consistency

Above everything, maintain consistency. The key to success is consistency. In the same way that you must regularly work on anything you do in your life to be successful, so must you work on your fitness objective. Consistency is essential for attaining any fitness objective, whether it is increasing muscle mass and strength, losing weight, or any other particular goal. To get the most out of your activities, you must put in consistent effort and stick to your training regimen.

Muscle development is often a slow and constant process that happens over time. Only by being constant can your stamina improve and your workouts become more effective and efficient. Resist making excuses for taking extended pauses from your exercises, even though you know in your heart that you don't. The first step toward achieving consistency is to establish a basic training plan, which we already have in Chapter 6. So, what do you think? You're already a long way from achieving consistency. A smart exercise schedule should keep you on track and in accordance with your training objectives.

The strategy for each workout is carefully laid out so that you do not have to worry about the exercises you will have to execute or what you will have to do in your next session.
A solid fitness regimen should also include activities that work the muscles throughout your body. That is exactly what my proposed solution in Chapter 6 accomplishes. But it is important to understand that even if you have the most efficient and flawless exercise plan in place, if you are unable to remain consistent and stick to it, it will not assist you in any way.
A number of things happen in your body while you workout. Your body goes through specific chemical processes and releases of chemicals (hormones) that cause changes in your body. The more

you exercise, the more responses and secretions occur in your body, causing it to alter and become more strong and efficient.

This implies that if you stick to your training routine, your body will adjust to the changes, allowing you to get stronger and perform better in your workouts.

When you practice hard activities on a regular basis, your muscles get damaged as a result of the training. This disturbs the organelles of your muscle cells, activating the satellite cells. The satellite cells are then triggered by your body's hormones, which cause your muscle fibers to grow in size.

We all want a physique that is strong, healthy, and attractive. Yet, you must recognize that you must embrace consistency in order to attain, if not all, at least one of these objectives. Make your exercise a habit if you want to be consistent with it. The more often you do the exercises, the more natural they become.

Things may seem difficult at first. You could even feel inclined to give up. But don't do it. Just remember that consistency is the key to unlocking success in your training objectives, and the rest will fall into place. That's all. Your body will adjust. In fact, you'll never want to skip a workout again. Yet, before you get there, you must focus on consistency. The more you exercise, the more your body will get used to it, and it will become more of a habit, if not a pastime.

Strategies for Maintaining Consistency

Prepare for setbacks. Consider all of the circumstances that can compel you to take longer pauses from working out and prepare for them. Take the initiative. We all face stumbling blocks in our everyday lives that might set us back or cause us to stumble. Having a strategy for overcoming these challenges prepares you both physically and mentally to go on. For example, if you have to attend infrequent gatherings after work, you may arrange your calendar so that your schedule is less stressful. You must also account for inclement weather and other timing restrictions.

Make use of reminders. When you first start doing anything new that isn't part of your regular routine, it's easy to forget to do it until it becomes a habit. You may forget that you need to exercise on a certain day. You may even forget that you are following an exercise routine at times. Set reminders on your phone, calendar, watch, or even smart assistants to prevent forgetting to exercise. You may also print your exercise plan and place it near your mirror, refrigerator, or office desk.

Negative ideas should be avoided. All achievement begins in the mind. What you believe is who you are. Most of us allow our brains to derail our plans and objectives. If you are familiar with the phrase "we are our own worst enemies," you will understand what I am referring to. If you are constantly thinking "I can't...", "I am not...", and other negative ideas, you are less likely to exercise regularly.

Be dedicated. Commitment entails doing something even if you don't want to do it, don't enjoy it, or it is inconvenient. Dedication is also a crucial factor in achieving success. To be successful in anything, you must be dedicated. As a result, if you want to establish consistency in your routine, you must commit to training for at least 30 days. Whether you exercise once a week, twice a week, or three times a week, doing it for a month will help you stick with it. Do you want to know why a month? According to research, it takes a typical human being 24 days of doing something repeatedly to form a habit.

Determine your objective. Focus more on short-term objectives. Some long-term ambitions may seem impractical and unattainable. Put out your aim and double-check it to verify it is SMART (specific, measurable, achievable, relevant, and time-limited). Relate it to something meaningful in your life so that it might take root deep inside you. Go the extra mile and explain the reasons for having such a goal, as well as the anticipated advantages after accomplishing the objective. Instead of setting a goal like "exercise regularly," set a goal like "exercise 2-3 days a week for 30 minutes for the next 18 weeks," since it will help you grow muscle mass and energy, take care of yourself, and play with your children.

Maintain a regular exercise schedule. Beginning a fitness quest without a training regimen is one of the most common reasons for failure. "What gets planned, gets done," as the saying goes. It's one thing to declare you'll exercise; quite another to really do it. When you schedule your exercise on your calendar or planner, it becomes more genuine. It also holds you responsible, keeps you on track, and makes exercise a priority.

Begin small and work your way up. Lifting larger weights and executing more sets and reps should be done gradually. Most individuals who stop exercising begin at a speed that they are unable to sustain for an extended period of time. Begin slowly and progressively increase the intensity of your exercise, sets, reps, and weight as you gain strength.

Please be patient. "Rome wasn't built in a day," you've surely heard. Muscles cannot be built overnight. Most individuals expect to see results immediatelyou've surely heard. Muscles cannot be built overnight. Most individuals expect to see results immediately. Such expectations are irrational. You must also be gentle with yourself if you find that you are not completely adhering to your fitness program. You must recognize that developing a new habit takes time. Just have faith in the process and be patient. Everything will fall into place.

Seek out responsibility. While others are watching, people are more inclined to stick to their training program. Find an accountability friend for yourself if you want to be completely dedicated to making changes. This person might be your partner, a friend, or a family member. Nobody wants to let down their exercise partner or someone they care about. When selecting an accountability partner, choose someone with whom you share a similar training routine and commit to it.

Maintain a record of your progress. Track your progress on a weekly basis to see how far you've come. Make a note of any progress you make. Viewing your accomplishments motivates you to workout more and improve in areas where you believe you are lacking.

Make exercising more pleasant. Try several techniques to make your training enjoyable. You may associate exercise with something fun, such as a game, take it outside and do it with friends, or reward yourself to encourage your consistent effort.

To obtain a healthier, stronger, fitter, and leaner physique, you must include exercise in your daily routine. When the recommendations above are carefully considered, they will assist you in staying consistent with your training and seeing long-term improvement.

Exercise Stagnation

Typically, our bodies will reach a point of stagnation. Exercise stagnation simply implies that you follow your training regimen religiously but observe no change or positive outcomes. Stagnation normally develops when your muscles adapt to a certain training regimen and the same stimulus on a regular basis. As a consequence, your exercise performance suffers, your muscles cease developing, and your body fails to record any muscle growth progress.

Exercise plateauing is a typical and natural occurrence. That occurs to everyone. If you haven't already, you will attain it as you exercise. When you hit a plateau in your exercise, you must adjust your plan and approach. What you should do is as follows:

Increase your sets and reps. If you've been doing three sets of six repetitions, try four sets of ten reps with less weight. Change your reps and sets as you develop to let your body adjust.

Warm up before you begin exercising. Warm up your muscles by doing some warm-up activities like running in place before beginning your workout.

Change your exercise regimen. Use alternate exercises from Chapter

4 to redefine and adjust your present training regimen. What we're aiming to accomplish here is work our muscles from various angles. This provides fresh triggers for muscular development in your body. Develop a nutrition plan that complements your exercise. Prepare a meal that will provide your body with the required energy and nutrients before and after your exercise.

Reduce your repeat pace. This allows your muscles to spend more time under stress, allowing them to move through their complete range of motion.

Attempt to do your workouts in less time than you thought. Doing more workouts in a shorter amount of time exposes your muscles to fresh stimuli, encouraging them to expand.

Strive for a balance of volume and intensity. Never ignore your body. If your exercise intensity is high, limit the number of sessions you undertake each week; if it is low, increase the number of sessions.

When you put your muscles through a specific level of activity, your body reacts by generating new muscles to deal with the circumstance. But, bear in mind that the demand on these forces is continual and recurrent, which means your body must constantly develop new muscles. This implies that you must be persistent with your workouts in order to help your muscles generate new strength to deal with stress.

When you acquire consistency, it is quite satisfying. On the other side, it is very irritating when you fail to attain it since you also fail to reach your objective.

You already know that you have to keep up with your workouts if you want to get the body shape you want or reach any other training goal.

It is also vital to understand that most individuals give up when confronted with consistency challenges, and you may be one of them. But you don't have to. You will miss out on the opportunity to reach your fitness goal. Just be gentle on yourself.

Remember that consistency is a talent that requires time to master. Just enduring all of the hurdles that come with working out will result in consistency.

Key Takeaways When it comes to achieving your strength training objectives, consistency is your most powerful weapon. Maintain consistency in your training routine, diet, and recuperation.

Conclusion

The many advantages of strength training cannot be overstated. Whatever your age, It is never too late to start. You should be aware that the much-touted muscle mass loss that happens after we reach the age of 30 intensifies when we remain physically inactive. Strength training may help you gain muscle mass, manage chronic conditions, increase bone strength and health, and do much more. If you want to be healthy, strong, and in shape, this book is for you.

If you've been following along, you should be aware that strength training is the best approach to reaching these three goals: a strong, healthy, and fit physique. If you're new to strength training, making this type of commitment may be scary since it takes you out of your comfortable comfort zone. Yet it is your only option if you want to reach this valuable aim. You will succeed if you approach it with the appropriate mentality!

Important Takeaways

You must discover the appropriate motivation for your strength training. Discover your fitness whys. You will be able to do whatever it takes to attain them if you do so. Making time for training may seem like a monumental endeavor, but if you plan wisely, you will have an excess of it. Begin your training gently and methodically. Establish sensible objectives and commit to working hard to achieve them. Remember that if you don't have a goal or destination in mind, you're more likely to fail. Consider one. Be patient as you begin your training. Good things take time, and attaining a strong, healthy, and fit physique is no exception. A bottle of good wine takes years to develop. So, please be patient!

Exercise does not require a lot of equipment. Strength training does not require the use of expensive or specialized weightlifting equipment or gym-style machinery. It is, nonetheless, a good idea to invest in a few items of equipment. There is inexpensive weight lifting equipment on the market that will serve you well. You don't have to spend a fortune on pricey equipment. You have everything you need with only one kettlebell to produce tremendous progress from your workout regimen without breaking the bank. You will discover that it is well worth your money, and you will never be sorry. While you may attain your strength training goals using just your body weight, I feel that utilizing free weights, particularly a kettlebell, is the most effective alternative.

Make a fitness schedule. Anyone who does not plan is planning to fail. I've created a fitness routine just for you. To get the maximum benefits from strength training, follow this regimen for at least four weeks. It will assist you in staying on track and training successfully. Maintain consistency, and remember to gradually stress your muscles with heavier weights, repetitions, or sets.

Maintain a healthy diet. Never underestimate the importance of diet in achieving your fitness objectives. Remember that your food may make or ruin your strength training exercise. Take caution with what you eat. This does not imply foregoing your favorite dishes in favor of bland ones. You can still exercise while eating the meals you like.

You must prioritize the nutrients that your body needs. If you don't get enough of them from your diet, you may take supplements. Nonetheless, I advise individuals to try to acquire all of their nutrients from real meals rather than supplements. On the other side, there are certain items that you should avoid, such as processed meals. Avoid sugary and processed meals since they will really harm your health.

It is advised that you eat 1.2–1.7 grams of protein per kilogram of your target body weight or 0.5–0.8 grams of protein per pound of your target body weight every day.

Consuming 20-40 grams of protein before and after your workout is suggested. Doing your exercises in supersets is the best way to save time while getting the most out of your workout.

To enjoy the advantages of both muscle and strength growth, you must execute three sets of six to twelve repetitions.
You must also workout 1-3 days each week, with rest days in between.

Exercising safely is important. Remember, the aim here is to maintain fitness, muscular mass, and strength as well as excellent health and avoid accidents. Make sure you exercise regularly. Don't push yourself too hard, too soon. Start small and gradually progress. While doing the motions, maintain appropriate form. It is critical that you be safe. Do not overwork your muscles. Provide ample time for them to recuperate.

Maintain consistency. Remember that persistence is your most powerful weapon in achieving your ideal physique.
Last, you must be well hydrated. To avoid dehydration, drink plenty of water before, during, and after exercise. Preferably, you should drink 8 glasses of water every day, which corresponds to 2 liters. Thus, drink at least 2 liters of water every day.
The most certain approach to reaching your fitness objectives is to combine strength training with adequate diet, recuperation, and hydration. Just be consistent and make sure to do your exercises carefully, and you will be pleased with the results.
Now that you have everything you need to develop a strong, fit, and healthy physique, go out and find it. You must put more effort into putting what you've learned in this book into practice; otherwise, the knowledge contained within will be trivial and impotent to transform your body and life. The most essential aspect of anyone's life is to have fun and be happy doing what they like. Strength training, as it is for me, should be one of those things.

Made in the USA
Coppell, TX
18 November 2024